JUGGLING
RHINOS

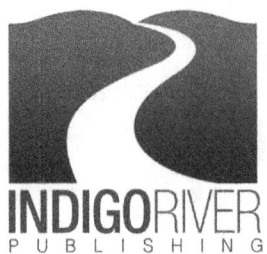

JUGGLING RHINOS

Finding Hope & Strength when Life's Problems are Charging Right at You

Kristy Geiser

JUGGLING RHINOS
Finding Hope & Strength when Life's Problems are Charging Right at You

Copyright © 2012 by Kristy Geiser

All rights reserved. No portion of this publication may be reproduced, stored in a retrieval system, or transmitted by any means—electronic, mechanical, photocopying, recording, or any other—except for brief quotations in printed reviews, without the prior written permission of the publisher.

All Scriptural references are from the King James Version of the Bible.

Editors: Adam Tillinghast, Donna Melillo

Cover Design: Jason Kauffman / Firelight Interactive / firelightinteractive.com

Interior Design: Tracie Maltezo

Indigo River Publishing
3 West Garden Street Ste. 352
Pensacola, FL 32502
www.indigoriverpublishing.com

Ordering Information:
Quantity sales: Special discounts are available on quantity purchases by corporations, associations, and others. For details, contact the publisher at the address above.

Orders by U.S. trade bookstores and wholesalers: Please contact the publisher at the address above.

Printed in the United States of America

Publisher's Cataloging-in-Publication Data is available upon request.

ISBN 978-0-9856033-0-4

First Edition

With Indigo River Publishing, you can always expect great books, strong voices, and meaningful messages. Most importantly, you'll always find... words worth reading.

Dedication

This book is dedicated to my Lord and Savior without Whom I would have no story.

Also to my wonderful husband, who has meant more to me than I could have ever hoped—my rock and support, my best friend, and the only one with whom I could imagine being by my side on this journey.

Table of Contents

Using Our Story to Get Through Yours 10

The Calm Before the Storm 12

Weathering the Storm 20

God Doesn't Make Mistakes 34

The Eye of the Storm 40

Lightning Strikes 46

Losing a Parent 50

Robbing Peter to Pay Paul 56

Learning from Job & Paul 64

Blessing in Disguise 70

A Time for Rejoicing 78

The Unexpected News 84

Another Go-Around 90

Preparing for the New Addition 98

Family of Three? 106

A Brave Little Girl 112

Holidays in Memphis 120

The Sun Shines Brighter 126

Lessons from Our Family 136

Sources of Inspiration 142

Epilogue: My Personal Message...................... 150

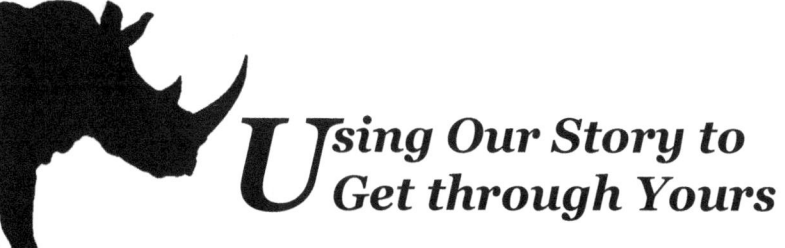
Using Our Story to Get through Yours

Using Our Story to Get through Yours

She has cancer—these words would come to shape our lives for many years to come. The doctor looked into Abby's eyes, and without a moment's hesitation, he said, "Abby has retinoblastoma—she has cancer..." No matter what his next words were, it didn't matter. I immediately thought, "No. Things like this don't happen to *me*! They only happen to *other* people." I never imagined that I would hear the words *my baby* and *cancer* in the same sentence. Those words came down on me like a load of bricks.

Honestly, there have been times when I felt my world crumbling all around me; but I have also felt God upholding me throughout those storms. If you find yourself at a place in your life where the waves are crashing all around you, and you feel like all hope is lost, please take heart. No matter what your storm—whether financial, the death of a loved one, a child with cancer, or one of many other difficulties—I want you to know that you have the opportunity to prosper and grow as you learn to trust God. In fact, I believe that is God's purpose for the storms in our lives. Whether you can relate to having a child with cancer or not, my hope is that there may have been other storms in my life that you *can* relate to that will help encourage you personally.

Although we don't choose to go through a storm or experience pain, we can look back and realize that we are actually stronger for having gone through them. My goal is to show you, through my family's story, that we can embrace storms as a crucial part of life to grow and give our life more meaning. We cannot escape storms in our lives, but we can allow them to help make us better.

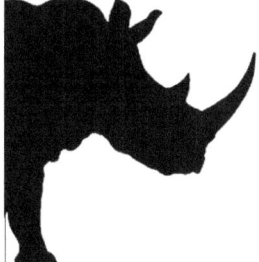

The Calm Before the Storm

The Calm Before the Storm

My life had always been pretty normal—fairly free of storms. I grew up in a normal, loving, Christian family. I went through life doing the normal things that people do: I went to school; I went to college; I got married; I had children—you know, "normal" things. Nothing much out of the ordinary really ever happened in my life.

The biggest problems I ever had to worry about while growing up were things like: what to wear to school, someone saying something mean to me, or having to change a dirty diaper when I babysat. My life was "packed" with homework, driver's education, and working a 20-hour a week job. (Oh, to have a worry-free life again!) Yes, this all sounds sarcastic—it is meant to be! But, this is very close to the truth. I had quite a worry-free life growing up.

Even into my early adult life, I didn't know much about weathering personal storms. I hadn't witnessed any—maybe because of the careful and loving protection of my parents while I grew up—I wasn't aware of the effects of life's storms. I didn't know about the fear associated with the unknown; my home had been virtually void of fear. I hadn't experienced heartache that was difficult to explain. I hadn't learned to fully rely on God for anything; I didn't have to rely on Him in my life free of storms.

When I graduated from college, I felt that the Lord wasn't moving me away just yet. I got a job at the college and was happily employed when I met Skip later that same year. During the time that we were dating and later engaged, I had no doubts that God had placed Skip into my life to be my husband, best friend, and soul-mate. He was the perfect man for me, and I was thankful for his godly character, which helped me grow in my own spiritual life. That is what I needed in a husband. After we got married, Skip started our family off on the right foot and has maintained that path for us as we've continued on.

Nine and a half months later, God blessed us with a

beautiful daughter, Emma Leigh, and our lives were just as perfect as any young couple blessed by their first child. She was absolutely precious and brought so much happiness and delight to our home. It was such an amazing feeling becoming a parent. I didn't realize how much love I could have for a child until Emma was born! We enjoyed watching all of her "firsts," and she amazed us as she seemed so advanced—to us anyway, as the biased parents. We were blissfully living the typical American life.

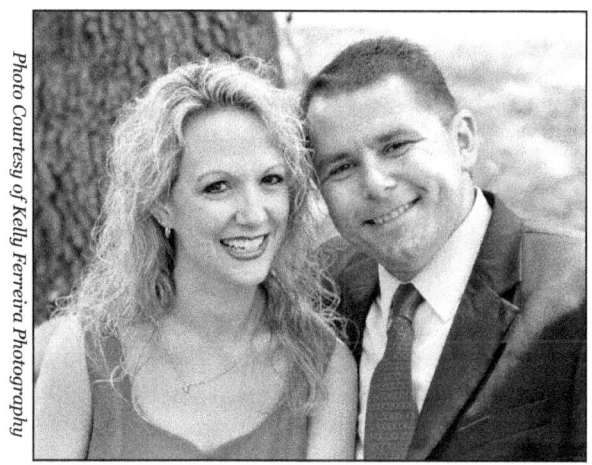

Skip (my husband and best friend) and I.

I was still employed when I had Emma, so when it came time for me to go back to work after my maternity leave, I had the most difficult time leaving her. An excellent nursery was provided, but I just felt horrible leaving her in the care of someone else. Skip and I decided then that I should stay home, now that I was a mother. We felt that the Lord didn't give us this child for someone else to rear, so after I finished my contract, I stayed home with her. I realized that staying home with Emma was the best decision we could have made. She and I enjoyed each other as we both learned so much—she about life, and I about parenting!

We enjoyed being the "perfect" little family, and within a

year, we purchased our first home—we were pretty much just like any other family we knew. Shortly after Emma turned one, we found out that we were expecting our second child. We were so excited about the new addition. I really hoped in my heart that it would be a girl, so Emma would have a little sister. I enjoyed my Emma, and I really liked the thought of having two daughters. Of course, when the ultrasound came about, I *had* to find out if it was a boy or a girl. To our delight, it *was* a girl! I was elated!

Abbigail Joy arrived just before Emma's second birthday. It had been a difficult birth, but she was perfect. I was so excited to have my two daughters. I just knew they would grow up being the best of friends—and of course, at times, the worst of enemies! Life was good, and I continued to enjoy being a stay-at-home mommy.

It was quite the adjustment going from one child to two. It took me a while to figure out how to juggle taking care of two children, especially when it came time to venture out of the house alone. For instance, what if I needed to take Emma to the restroom while we were in the store? What would I do with Abby? After figuring it all out, we settled into a routine, and everything just became second nature.

I was also, however, beginning to realize that storms are a part of life. We all have them, obviously with varying intensity. No one escapes life without going through storms—whether spiritual, physical, or emotional. At this time, I was waking up and realizing that life wouldn't always be as perfect as it had seemed.

About six weeks after Abby's birth, I went to my obstetrician for my postpartum checkup. After the routine tests, I found out my results came back abnormal. I wondered what that could mean for me and my future. Because my sister had borderline cervical cancer a year or so before, and my family has a pretty heavy history of cancer, I was a little concerned about these results. The follow-up test would be a couple of months down the road.

Over the next few weeks, the strangest thing happened. All of a sudden, I started hearing message after message, and reading scripture after scripture, about storms in our lives. Suddenly, it seemed *every* preacher was preaching about Job! They told of his horrible trials; they spoke of how Job remained faithful throughout his storms. They taught about trials and tribulations that we will face and how God can use them in our lives. Each of them was preaching about how we should respond, as Christians, when these trials come.

God had my attention! I *knew* He had prepared those words for *me*. There was no doubt that these were things I was *supposed* to hear. It seemed more than just a coincidence that I was hearing all of this during one short period of time. It could only mean that He just *had* to be preparing my heart for an upcoming storm.

My mind began to whirl. What would my prognosis be? What would this mean for my husband and two small daughters? My girls were too young to understand what Mommy would be going through. How difficult would it be for us to endure this trial that was coming up?

The follow-up test came about, and in my heart, I was prepared to hear negative results. After all, *God had been speaking to me directly about this!* He had all but told me Himself, in an audible voice, that I had cancer. But to my surprise, my test results came back just fine—nothing abnormal. Everything was within normal limits. I didn't have cancer! Oh, the relief that came from those test results.

I was so confused. I had been *sure* that God had been preparing my heart by letting me know that He was there to take care of whatever valley He would take me through. All I had to do was trust in Him. Why then had I been bombarded by messages from the Lord about an upcoming trial in my life?

Little did I know that my answer would come a few weeks later. Abby's four-month checkup had been scheduled, and Skip and I took her on a Thursday toward the end of September to the pediatrician's office. I had previously wondered about her eyes because, when she would look at a distance, her left eye would wander and wouldn't track the same as her right eye. We mentioned this to the pediatrician, and as he inspected her eyes, he said that we should take her to an ophthalmologist for further consultation. He said there was only one pediatric ophthalmologist in our area, and nonchalantly said I should take her to see him in the next week or so. Well, that was the plan: we would call them to set up an appointment for Abby to see if there was anything wrong with her eyes.

A little later that same afternoon, the ophthalmologist's office called me and told me they had an opening early the next morning, and that they could see Abby. Looking back, it is strange that it never occurred to us that this may be an indication that something serious could be wrong.

Skip decided to take some time off work to go with me because his curiosity was piqued as to how they would examine a four-month-old's eyes. This was amazing in and of itself, because Skip rarely went to the kids' doctor's appointments with me; but, thankfully, he had gone with me that week to Abby's appointments. Skip and I had been thinking that Abby might have a lazy eye and would probably need to wear an eye patch or something. There was not even a thought in either of our minds that it could possibly be anything serious.

Well, Friday morning came, and Skip and I took our little Abby to the eye doctor. After the normal doctor's office routine, we were called back. The doctor looked into her eyes and, without a moment's hesitation, said, "Abby has retinoblastoma—she has cancer..." No matter what his next words were, it didn't matter. These three words—*she has cancer* (every parent's fear)—would be the words that would come to shape our lives for many years to come.

What a blow this news was to us! My initial reaction was, "What? No! Things like this *don't* happen to *me!* They only happen to *other* people." He continued to explain that tumors in her eyes were causing them to not track the same way. She had a large tumor in the back of her left eye, which was blocking its vision. In a typical doctor tone, he abruptly prepared us for the fact that Abby would need to see a specialist; this was not something that he could treat. Because there weren't any specialists in our area, we would have to travel for the help and treatments she would need.

He said she would receive chemotherapy and would need to have her eye removed. The doctor was preparing us for what was to come—for the future events we would have to face. That caused us a great amount of trepidation about our future, which would now include these completely unfamiliar circumstances.

Chemotherapy seemed like an awful proposition to us. Abby was just a baby—this was *our baby* we were talking about! How could we do this to her? And to have her eye removed seemed deplorable! However, we knew there was no option other than to have her treated if we wanted her to live.

Our minds were reeling. We had stepped foot in that doctor's office on just a regular Friday morning, and stepped out into a journey that would carry us past our natural limits. Where would we go from there?

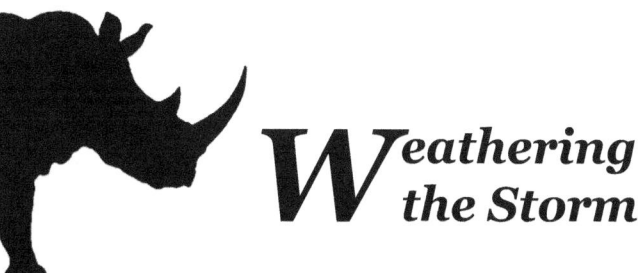

Weathering the Storm

Weathering the Storm

I can still vividly remember the feeling I had as I walked away from the doctor's office with four-month-old Abby in my arms. I can see the path I walked as tears welled in my eyes and spilled down my cheeks. I felt so overwhelmed and helpless. I felt weak knowing that I couldn't fix this for her like I so desperately longed to. After all, that is what mothers do. They kiss the boo-boos and make them better. How could I make this one better for her? Words cannot fully describe my feelings that morning!

Here I found myself, holding this beautiful child whom I loved so desperately, knowing that she now had such a tough road ahead of her. She would have to face things that seem unimaginable for such a young child. Why her? Why not me? I was supposed to be the one going through the storm, not my sweet, tiny baby girl!

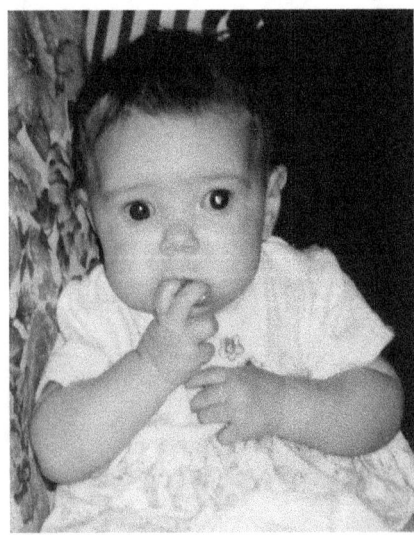

The effect on Abby's eyes was visible, even before her diagnosis.

I felt so inadequate, but I hoped I would be able to give Abby all the love and support she would need as she went through this life-changing ordeal. All I could do was hold her as tightly as I could, and hope that I could be the loving, comforting mother that she would need in the months and years ahead.

As we drove home, we were numb, in shock, and perhaps maybe even in a little bit of denial. What do we do now? We were suddenly the parents of, medically, a very needy child! How does a family function with a child who has cancer? What challenges does a child face without one of her eyes? How would she cope, and what ridicule would she have to endure as a child? As I thought of our impending journey, I was thankful to realize that Abby was young enough to not remember much, if anything, of what she would have to go through.

It was encouraging to see God's hand beginning to work in the details of our situation. I can't imagine how difficult it would have been to tell Skip the doctor's news myself! How do you break that type of news to anyone—especially someone as close as your spouse? God was gracious in that we were able to hear the diagnosis together!

We made it home, and I remember sitting at the dining room table just crying. I was absolutely miserable and in shock about the news we had just learned about our baby. I wasn't sure if I even wanted to *try* to sort things out in my mind. We knew there was so little we could do for Abby as this awful disease was invading her tiny body. At this point, we didn't know the details of the prognosis of a child with retinoblastoma. We tried to not let our minds think the worst, but it is almost impossible when cancer is brought into the picture.

Skip had taken it as hard as I had, and at first, all we could do was just pray, cry, and sit in silence. There weren't any words that either of us could say. We just couldn't wrap our minds around the fact that *our* baby had cancer! How could this be? I had never even heard of anything like this. We learned that retinoblastoma is a rare disease: about 300 children are diagnosed with retinoblastoma each year in the United States. We were totally taken aback with what we had just learned about our daughter's illness.

Our lives were *completely* turned upside down. Nothing would be the same—at least not for a very long time. In order to get our child well, we knew we had no choice but to follow the path we had suddenly found ourselves on.

We wished there was an option to bargain with God to take this awful disease from Abby and give it to us; either of us could go with only one eye, but not our little girl! As her parents, we wanted Abby to have the best possible chances in life, not the limitations associated with her disease and impending treatment.

Whether we liked it or not, we had to pursue treatment, no matter how grim it seemed. After receiving the devastating news earlier that day, we had asked the ophthalmologist which hospital he would take his child to if he were in our shoes. He directed us to St. Jude Children's Research Hospital in Memphis, Tennessee. His office immediately contacted them for us, and we were contacted by St. Jude's staff that same afternoon to set up our schedule. This schedule would require an immediate trip, the first of *many*, to Memphis. We were told that we needed to act quickly to get Abby's treatment started because of the seriousness of Abby's condition.

Skip and I struggled briefly with the decision of whether or not to allow chemotherapy as a treatment for Abby. Having to make such a drastic, life-changing decision for your child is a complicated and difficult proposition. As soon as the news began to spread, some well-meaning friends warned us against giving her chemo because of the harsh effects on the body. We were at a loss! As we researched *natural* remedies, we found that they would likely take eighteen months or more to work—even then, there was no guarantee. Because this disease is so aggressive, Abby didn't have that much time if she were to have a chance to keep her eyes. Natural or traditional treatments—both have pros and cons. To us, the chemo seemed the lesser of two evils, and we both felt a peace that this would be the best option for Abby.

Many wonderful people rallied around us as the news spread of Abby's diagnosis. There were several who offered their help with whatever we needed. It was difficult to tell them, since we really didn't know what we needed ourselves. However, we knew they cared and would be there if we did need them. There were others who offered prayer for Abby and for us—we were so thankful for our godly friends and family who prayed for us. There were also many who offered gifts of food or money to help with travel and other expenses—that was also a tremendous help and very much appreciated.

People were so kind, and we were at a loss as to how to respond to the sudden attention. We were extremely thankful for the love and support that was shown to us. God used so many people to be a blessing to us during those first days after Abby's diagnosis.

We decided to go ahead and drive most of the way to Memphis on Saturday, so we could get away and be alone with our thoughts. The four of us stopped at a hotel overnight and continued on to Memphis on Sunday, where we were provided housing. We ended up at St. Jude Children's Research Hospital the following Monday morning, September 30, 2002, for our appointments. It had been such a whirlwind going from a "normal" life on Thursday to finding ourselves in Memphis on Monday! Thursday we were at a normal checkup at the pediatrician; Friday we were at the eye doctor; and Monday we were in appointments at St. Jude Children's Research Hospital.

Despite our circumstances, I'll never forget the amazing feeling of peace I had from Saturday on. I had spent Friday trying futilely to sort everything out in my mind—what had just happened, what to do, and where to go from here. On Saturday, I somehow truly felt a peace that surpassed my human understanding. I could already see God's hand working in the situation; all I had to do was rely on Him.

Throughout the next two weeks in Memphis, the Lord flooded my heart with such a peace. He showed me that He had Abby in His hand. He removed the anxiety and gave me the assurance that He would take care of her. He had a plan for her life, which included her present circumstances. He brought back things I had heard in those messages about living through the storms that helped me immensely! No more tears were shed over her newly found diagnosis—peace took over!

The schedule of those two weeks brought a barrage of appointments, including several scans, surgery to insert a central line into her chest, her first dose of chemotherapy, and many other tests. She was poked and prodded so many times; this is always difficult for a mother to witness! Watching such a small child getting prepared for and going under anesthesia seems so abnormal. One can't help but think that they are too small to be going through such medical procedures, but these were all steps we had to take in order for her to get well.

It was a little unsettling when we saw our little baby come out of surgery with her central line. It looked so anomalous. At first, we just saw a bandage with a tube sticking out of it; but when it came time for the bandage change, it was very unnerving to see such a malformation with a white tube coming out of the skin on her chest. We knew it had value, but that didn't make us feel much better. It was something new that we would have to get used to over the next few months. It would become a major focus, as it would require so much care as long as she had it.

The surgeons had to "thread" the central line through the artery in Abby's neck down through her chest, where it came out in the middle—a very precise surgery. During this surgery, they missed the artery on the right side, so they had to try again by going in the left side to place the line. In missing the right side, they touched a nerve, causing her eye to droop considerably. As she was waking up from her surgery, they explained this to us. They said that it might be permanent damage, but it might not be if they just "disturbed" it. If that was the case, it would go back to normal after a little while.

We were hopeful that this droop in her eye was just temporary damage, and that she wouldn't have this deformity throughout her life, adding to her other complications. Thankfully, after a few days, the damage was reversed and her eye started looking normal again. This brought to mind how our amazing bodies, thanks to our Creator, can heal such disturbances. A short time later, her eye looked just fine.

After Abby's first exam under anesthesia to look at her eyes, the doctors informed us that Abby had a very large tumor on the back of her left eye, as well as two smaller peripheral tumors. She also had six small peripheral tumors in her right eye.

Without having a medical background, here is how it sounded to me as the doctor educated us about Abby's disease, helping answer the question of *how* she developed retinoblastoma:

Abby had a tiny mutation in her genes that altered her RB gene (which we know is God's design for her). She now had a defect in this gene because of the mutation. The RB gene is known to be a major cancer suppressor. Only one of the two chromosomes on this "rung" of her DNA can fight cancer, so they prepared us that Abby would be prone to cancer throughout her life. She could have up to five different cancers throughout her lifetime.

As I had mentioned earlier, only about 300 children are diagnosed with retinoblastoma each year in the United States; of those 300 diagnoses, only about one case in four involve both eyes. Because she had this mutation, tumors showed up in both eyes. This was an indicator that her cancer is the *genetic* form of the disease. They completed a genetic test on us. While neither Skip nor I was found to be carriers of this gene, Abby had the mutation, causing the cancer in her eyes.

Since Abby carries the genetic form of retinoblastoma, any children Abby may have will have a 50 percent chance, or better, of having the same genetic defect, allowing retinoblastoma. What a struggle that could cause in the future—to have children or not, knowing they could likely be born with retinoblastoma! That would be a whole different discussion for another day.

Retinoblastoma can come in three forms: unilateral, bilateral, and trilateral. Unilateral retinoblastoma is only found in one eye and is usually *not* hereditary. Bilateral is found in both eyes and is generally hereditary. This is what Abby was diagnosed with. Retinoblastoma is considered trilateral when it has spread to the brain as well. If left untreated, Abby's cancer would have most likely spread to her brain next.

Fortunately, the doctors felt that they had developed an effective plan to treat Abby's cancer with chemotherapy. Because of the rapid progression of Abby's cancer, her tumors had formed "seeds," raising the concern that additional tumors could form in her eyes—or even in her brain. The doctors were fairly confident that chemotherapy would kill those seeds.

We were informed that retinoblastoma is inoperable because the tumors are *inside* the eye wall. Pressure cannot be restored in the eyeball once it is punctured; the only way to remove the tumors is by removing the eye. This is why the pediatric ophthalmologist had prepared us that they would most likely remove her eye.

Thankfully, the doctors at St. Jude decided *not* to remove her eye. They felt the best thing for Abby would be to see how she would do with chemotherapy and focal treatments, which included laser therapy and cryotherapy (freezing the tumors). They did prepare us, however, that she would never regain full vision in her left eye, and that there *could* be a time in the future that Abby may lose one entirely. In fact, for many children with retinoblastoma, this is a very common prognosis.

We were also thankful for our primary oncologist who cared so much for Abby and our family. God is so good at placing the right people in our lives at the right time to help us through difficult circumstances. Her doctor was one of those people. You knew he was there because he loved kids and wanted to help them. He was so good with Abby; the love and care he showed for her helped us to be confident that he would only do what was best for her.

The time was nearing that we were going to be able to go home, and we were so pleased that Abby would be able to keep both of her eyes for the time being! They taught us how to care for her at home and how to carry out her protocol. We were instructed that we would need to go back to Memphis every three weeks in order for Abby to receive chemotherapy. Every six weeks (every other visit), she would also have an exam under anesthesia where they would monitor the progress of the tumors.

When they were sending us home for the first time, I was completely overwhelmed at the thought of being Abby's nurse and taking care of her at home. At the hospital, everything was taken care of so well by trained professionals. While they trained me in caring for her, I wondered how I would be able to follow through with all the things I would have to do.

I would need to go through several steps to draw up the

medicine and flush her line each day. Abby's dressing would need to stay dry, and I would need to do dressing changes a couple times each week, which entailed several steps. Her line absolutely could not ever be submersed in water, which made bath time tricky. She needed her oral medications and the medicine for her eyes. She would need to be taken to the clinic twice a week to get blood drawn to make sure she wouldn't need blood transfusions. I would also need to keep her in a clean, almost sterile environment, clear of sickness and bacteria, since she would now be so prone to infection. I am definitely not a nurse, and this was all totally new to me!

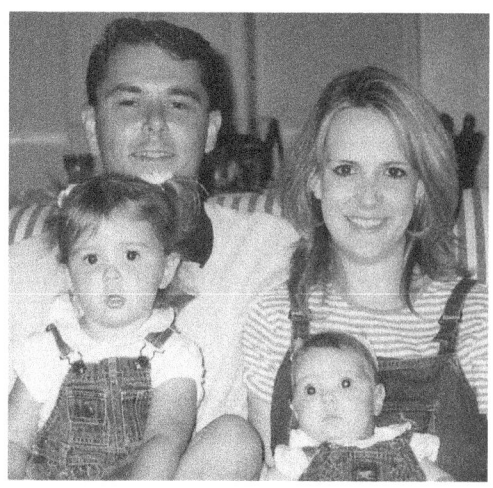

Our two beautiful girls.

The most nerve-racking thing was that I needed to do everything exactly right. There was so much that needed to be done for my baby girl. What if I missed a step? Or what if I forgot to do something important one day? When you are suddenly thrown into something so unfamiliar and detailed, it is daunting.

It ended up not being as much of a challenge as I thought, once I adjusted to my new way of life, adding Abby's medical care to my routine.. At the time, however, it definitely felt like an overwhelming proposition to me. Despite my fears, the Lord was with me and helped me take care of her. Soon, all of this became second nature to me, and my fear of taking care of her subsided.

Throughout the next six months, Abby was on two chemotherapy drugs: carboplatin and vincristine. Carboplatin is a cousin to another drug that is known to cause hearing loss.

Because of this, Abby had routine hearing tests to watch for any hearing change. This, other typical side effects, and even additional *possible* side effects, remained a concern in the back of our minds as we continued her treatment. What would be the long-term effects of her chemotherapy? How would her little body withstand the harsh drugs that were required to kill the cancer cells?

After just a few treatments, Abby's tumors had shrunk significantly and were becoming calcified. Her doctors were confident that the chemo was working exactly as it should, and they were pleased with how quickly it was working. Instead of being shaped like a ball as they were at the beginning (kind of popcorn-shaped), the tumors were now flattened and somewhat broken up. We were so thankful for how well Abby was doing! God's hand had been evident in the remarkableness of how her situation was unfolding. She had been able to keep both eyes, which was a blessing in and of itself.

Throughout those six months, we had to deal with the effects of the chemo on Abby's little body. The drugs made her sick, and all we could do was keep her as comfortable as possible. They gave us medicine to keep her side-effects to a minimum, helping considerably. She lost her hair; this was so sad for me because she actually *had* hair as a baby. She also didn't gain much weight, as would be expected with the nausea, vomiting, and loss of appetite associated with chemo.

There were also times that we had to take Abby to the hospital for blood transfusions, as her platelet counts dropped dangerously low. One time, I remember getting a call telling me that Abby's platelet count was down to 6,000 (normal is around 200,000), and that I should take her to the emergency room as soon as possible. We hurried and took her in, and I prayed that she wouldn't bleed to death on the way. It was scary to know that her platelet count was that low! Since then, I've realized that while that *is* dangerously low, the likelihood of her bleeding to death wasn't as high as I had feared. At the time, being the worried mother, I was in tears fearing the worst.

It was difficult being on the roller coaster that we were on.

We would deal with the sickness and side effects of the chemo, and then we would be relieved when she started feeling better. However, we knew that we would have to go back and do it all over again. It was so emotionally taxing, and we felt horrible for putting her through this. Having a baby on chemotherapy is traumatic—it is so difficult to see such a tiny child suffering through the terrible effects. But God continued to be faithful, and He freely and abundantly gave us enough grace to make it through each day, one at a time.

Fevers were another issue we faced during this time. They have to be taken very seriously in those children whose immune systems are compromised by chemo, since they have little or no ability to fight infection or sickness. Just by having a central line, which can harbor and grow bacteria without proper sterile procedures, cancer patients have an increased likelihood for infection. Often, fevers are the first sign of such infections.

Since Abby was on chemotherapy, a fever sent us immediately to the emergency room to check for an infection. The chemo causes the immune system to fail because it kills many of the "good" cells as well as the cancerous cells. The neutrophil cells are good cells that are depleted by the chemo. Neutrophils are the defense cells that fight off disease and bacteria. When the neutrophil counts are low, an infection can travel very quickly throughout the body if not treated right away by antibiotics.

Unfortunately, Abby was one of those babies who got a fever when she was teething. I know doctors say babies don't get a fever when they are teething, but that is the only explanation I had for her fevers. It seemed more than a coincidence that a fever came every time she was getting a new tooth. Regardless, every time she got a fever, I had to take her to the hospital for treatment; and each time, the fever was unexplained. It was somewhat frustrating because even though I suspected the fever was caused by her teething, it still needed to be taken seriously *in case* of an infection.

Because she received her chemotherapy throughout the winter, the infamous cold and flu season, we also had the fear of her being exposed to other sickness while we were visiting the emergency room. There were so many things to watch for. We were, however, grateful to know that if she were to get sick, it wouldn't catch God by surprise. It would only be because He allowed it. She was amazingly healthy throughout that winter, for which we were very thankful.

We had spent so much time in hospitals throughout those months—between the visits to St. Jude, lab draws twice a week, in-patient hospital stays for blood transfusions, and emergency room visits. By the end of her treatments in March of 2003, it was such a relief to be able to only have to go back to St. Jude every six weeks for checkups to be sure the tumors in her eyes remained stable. She continued to do very well, with only occasional local treatments when a concern would arise that one of her tumors wasn't "acting right."

During our visit to Memphis in October 2003, Abby was able to have her central line removed! It was such a blessing to not have to deal with the care and risks associated with her having it. It had been a huge help in her care, but we were ready to see it go! Now she could bathe and swim without the risk of getting her chest wet. What a great feeling after having the restrictions and care of a central line for over a year. It also sealed in our minds that her treatments were complete!

A moderate scar remains where Abby had her central line. The scar helps us remember the lessons of God's goodness to us throughout this time. Many times, God allows scars in our lives to remain as a gentle reminder of His faithfulness.

Our biggest praise was that Abby was still with us. Secondly, she had still been able to retain both of her natural eyes. We did know that they could do amazing things with prosthetic eyes; but thankfully, that was one less worry to think about. We would have to be cautiously optimistic that Abby would be able to keep both of her eyes.

When we were in Memphis during one of our first visits, I remember meeting another St. Jude mother on the elevator in the hotel where we were staying. She was there with her daughter, who was wearing an eye patch. The daughter was six years old and had just lost one of her eyes to retinoblastoma a week or so before. I remember her mother telling me that they had been hoping that she would be the first retinoblastoma patient to be able to keep both of her eyes. I'm not sure if she was correct in that every other child with retinoblastoma, six and over, has lost at least one eye, but it did make a pretty big impact on me at the time.

Despite my earlier fears of inadequacy, the Lord continued to sustain us through it all, and we felt His hand guiding and protecting us as we continued along our journey. Abby's little body took a beating with the harsh drugs, but little by little she strengthened. Over time, Abby's visits to St. Jude finally spread out to every six months. This valley then appeared to be a struggle of the past, and our days seemed brighter as we regained some sense of normalcy.

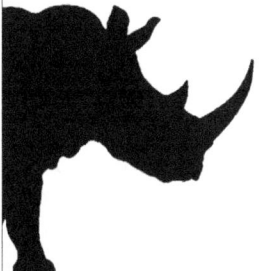
God Doesn't Make Mistakes

God Doesn't Make Mistakes

What could possibly be the purpose for this storm? Did the Lord make a mistake when He formed Abby? How could He have *allowed* this tiny mutation in her genes—the one causing my baby to have cancer? Some may say that this must be a mistake. A good and gracious God just couldn't allow something so terrible!

I couldn't help but wonder what God's plan is for Abby. This brought to my mind the story of her birth. Just a few days before Abby was born, Skip and I were invited to visit some friends at a beach house they rented while visiting our area. We had a great time visiting them, but while I was there, I ate some pretty spicy sausage. That night, in the middle of the night, I awoke to the feeling of Abby churning and churning inside—which I attributed to a probable reaction to the sausage I had eaten earlier.

I referenced earlier the difficulty of Abby's birth. Her birth was impeded because the cord was wrapped around her neck three times, holding her inside despite my efforts. I couldn't help but wonder if Abby's rolling movement a couple of nights before caused the umbilical cord to wrap around her neck. Finally, after about an hour of effort, she arrived miraculously without a cesarean. The doctor who delivered her stated, "Well, that's why she wouldn't come out; she was bungee jumping!" She safely cut the cord from around her neck, and I finally had my beautiful baby girl, seemingly healthy despite the circumstances. The doctor had kept a relaxed composure, and I was thankful for her calm manner, so as to not unduly upset or worry me. My mom lost her first baby because the umbilical cord had wrapped around the baby's neck. This had always been an underlying fear of mine when it came to the birth of my babies.

Why didn't our all-knowing God take Abby from us then, sparing her and us, from the treatments and hardships that she would have to endure in the coming months and years? As the cord was wrapped around her neck, He knew that she had retinoblastoma, yet He still gave her the blessing of life. Isaiah 44:2 says, "Thus saith the Lord that made thee, and formed thee from the womb, which will help thee." God wasn't surprised by the fact that Abby had cancer. He doesn't *ever* get taken by surprise. He had formed her in my womb, knowing that she would be born with this disease. God made Abby just the way He planned, and He is the only One who *could* give her the help she needed. This has proven to be true over and over as we realize our weaknesses. I can definitively say that Abby, or even her disease, was *not* a mistake by God. God doesn't make mistakes. Every being He forms *can* be used to glorify Him.

It is obvious that God has allowed this storm in her life. Did God allow this as an act of punishment or unkindness? Not at all. John 9 tells the story of a blind man. "And his disciples asked him, saying, Master, who did sin, this man, or his parents, that he was born blind? Jesus answered, Neither hath this man sinned, nor his parents, but that the works of God should be made manifest in him." Sometimes God allows storms in our lives to help draw us closer to Him, allowing us to be a testimony to others by sharing how God helped us through the hard times.

It's clear that God does have a plan for Abby, and He didn't allow this storm as an act of punishment. Abby was given to us for a reason. Abby was born as part of God's plan to draw us closer to Him and to teach us so much about Himself. In doing this, God gave us the ability to share with others the wonderful attributes of God. Abby was born to bring glory and honor to the Lord through her life, as each of us are, in reality.

We know from the Word of God that He is *good*, and only allows *good* things in the lives of His children. Romans 8:28 assures us, "And we know that all things work together for good to them that love God, to them who are the called according to his purpose." We can know that *all things*, even the storms and trials in our lives, work together for our good. God gives us that promise if we love Him! And Psalm 119:67-68, 71 says (emphasis mine), "Before I was afflicted I went astray, but now have I kept thy word. Thou art *good*, and doest *good;* teach me thy statutes. It is *good* for me that I have been afflicted, that I might learn thy statutes." Storms are learning experiences, often teaching us specifically of His kindness and love.

How can anyone consider afflicting a child with cancer to be *good?* First, Isaiah 55:8-9 tells us, "For my thoughts are not your thoughts, neither are your ways my ways, saith the Lord. For as the heavens are higher than the earth, so are my ways higher than your ways, and my thoughts than your thoughts." In other words, we cannot understand the mind of God; many times, these situations don't tend to make sense in our minds. Once we realize this, it is easier to trust an all-knowing God. Proverbs 3:5-6 states, "Trust in the Lord with all thine heart; and lean not unto thine own understanding. In all thy ways, acknowledge him, and he shall direct thy paths."

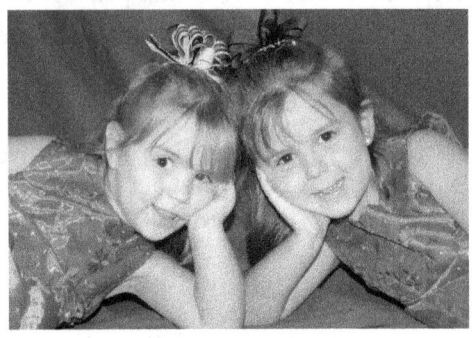
Our two blessings (Abby, left; Emma, right)

We need to give the storm to the Lord and let Him work. If we allow Him to work His perfect will, we will be blessed to see the end result. Those who try to oppose God or blame Him for their circumstances rob themselves of the joy and blessings that can be a result of giving the storm to Him. Seeing God's hand work through a storm is a wonderful way to experience God's power, grace, and goodness.

There are often times that we may give the situation to the Lord; but our tendency is to pick it back up at a later point, possibly when we don't feel He is working it out according to *our* plan and to our satisfaction. We need to let Him take care of it and work the situation out according to *His* plan so He may receive the honor and glory for what He has done.

His desire is for us to be able to come through the storm stronger and better individuals, but we need to allow Him free rein. After all, who knows better? Do we, or does the God of eternity? He can make anyone a stronger, better person and bring him closer to Himself through these trials. Abby is proof that God's goodness *can* come even from less-than-desirable circumstances. The storm gives us the ability to experience so many blessings that wouldn't otherwise be possible.

Even before we knew what joy she would bring to our family, we named her Abbigail Joy. Naming a second daughter is difficult—at least it was in our case. Naming Emma was easy. It was a name that we both liked from the start, and we were able to choose it almost immediately. When it came to naming our second daughter, we had already used the "easy" name, so we had to find yet another name that we both liked and could agree upon. After going through names for quite some time, we decided to name her Abbigail Joy simply because we thought it was a good name that we could both agree on, and we liked it because it was biblical. We also liked the meaning. Abbigail means "Father's Joy," so we have always thought of her as our double dose of Joy. She has been just that.

Even through difficult circumstances, we can look to the Lord for His help. God has the power to calm the wind and waves of a storm, but He also has the power to allow the storm to continue to crash in while calming His child. Even if He allows the storms to rage, we can still be thankful that He is upholding us in the palm of His hand, sustaining us through it all.

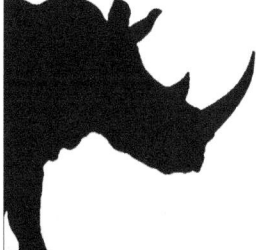

The Eye of the Storm

The Eye of the Storm

So, having a baby with retinoblastoma was our storm. That was the event God would use in our lives to bring Him glory. We were done. The rest of our lives would be wonderful—no more storms! Not in the least! God has continued to take us through the valleys and over the mountaintops.

As Abby's appointments continued to spread out, we had become a pretty normal family again. Cancer had ceased to be the center of our lives, and we went about our business as a typical family of four.

When she was a toddler, Abby did have a few issues with learning to compensate for her depth perception problems, due to having vision in only one eye. I remember almost crying once, as I watched my poor baby "miss" a curb, but that challenge was nothing she couldn't overcome with God's help. She eventually adapted to her disability. Abby has developed wonderfully, and has even excelled in pretty much every area, despite her circumstances. She is so smart, and has kept up with all of the other children her age.

Skip and I had known from the beginning of our marriage that we wanted a larger family, and we desired to have four children. I had thoroughly enjoyed my two girls and all that goes along with having daughters; so when I discovered in June of 2003 that we were expecting another child, I decided I would be happy with another girl. I also thought it would be neat, however, to have a boy. I didn't have any brothers, so I thought it would be a new and exciting experience for me to add a boy to our family. Either way, though, I wanted my last two to be the same gender, whether that be boys or girls.

God again added to our family by giving us our son, Micah James, in February 2004. Micah blessed us in such an amazing way, and I was immediately able to discover the joy that a son can bring to a mother's life. He was such a precious, laid-back boy who added so much to our family. He started out so tiny, but he grew and grew and stayed at the top of the height and weight chart. He is still so happy, can easily bring about a smile, and absolutely loves everyone he meets. I am so thankful that I am the mother of such a sweet and special boy!

Around the time of Micah's birth, Skip and I felt that the Lord was leading us in a different direction for Skip's career—to start a real estate business. It was a difficult decision because we had been so happy where we were, but it would be nice to be able to work out of the home together and have Skip be a bigger part of our lives. The Lord blessed us, and that quickly confirmed in our minds that this was the right move.

A little earlier than we had planned, but happily, I found out in October 2004 that I was expecting our fourth child. Micah was only eight months when we found out the news of the upcoming arrival. Now, because of the closeness in age of Micah and the new one to come, I desired our new bundle to be a boy. I thought it would be great, since they would essentially be one year apart, that they could grow up together as close brothers.

So, of course, I was excited about the ultrasound and finding out the gender of our little one. It was neat to see that God gave me what I hoped for—my last two would be boys. Zachariah William joined our family in May of 2005, just 15 months after Micah was born. Zach has proven to be our rambunctious little one who is "all-boy." He has been a blessing and has attached himself to Daddy and Mommy—he's happy just to be wherever we are. It has been great to see the boys grow together, being so close in age, because they are the best of friends. They do everything together—even pester the girls.

So, that rounded out our "perfect family" that we had planned. We now had the four children that we knew we wanted from the beginning. It was just perfect; we had two of each. Life was good, and each child brought something different to the family. Each personality has proven to be unique, and each child is not at all like any of the others. It has been eye-opening to see how God makes each of us special. Even with the same parents and the same upbringing, each child has his own special talents and attributes, and they are so vastly and distinctly diverse!

What a crazy time! I now had a four-year-old, three-year-old, one-year-old, and a newborn! Skip's philosophy had been, "Get 'em in, get 'em out." He wanted to have them, raise them, and then have time to retire with an empty nest, yet be young enough to enjoy each other and our grandchildren. We were well on our way toward that goal. I had my two baby boys as well as my two "big" girls. (Emma turned five a little over a month after Zach was born.) I enjoyed my children and never had a dull moment.

Because real estate is extremely busy during the summers, and we had four little ones to entertain, every moment of the day held a task for both Skip and me. Sleeplessness and busyness caused my memory to fail; needless to say, that summer is a blur in my mind. I guess this was somewhat of a blessing in disguise.

Later that year, in August of 2005, we found out what it was like to have a child in school. Emma started kindergarten that year, beginning our next chapter of parenting. It came up all of a sudden, and it was difficult for me once I realized my "baby girl" was old enough to go to school. She did well and enjoyed her time in class. It was during Emma's kindergarten year that her heart was pricked as her teacher was telling a Bible story, and Emma accepted Jesus Christ as her Savior.

We happily lived as a "normal" family who just happened to have a child with, now almost undetectable, cancer. Most people we came across didn't even know about the storm that we had weathered just a couple of years earlier.

Abby joined Emma in school the next year, in 2006, when she began K-4. We were then left with just the two boys at home in the mornings. This began our five-year stretch of picking up our children from school at both noon and three o'clock, and helped us to realize the value in car-pooling!

Our real estate business continued to do well, and we increased our business considerably throughout those first two and a half years. In July 2006, we were able to move into a larger home. With four children, we had quickly outgrown our three-bedroom home. When an opportunity came for us to purchase a bigger home, we decided to make the move.

In February 2007, we were able to go on a long-awaited trip that we were granted through Make-A-Wish for Abby. Of course, at the age of four, her "wish" was to go to Disney World. After months of preparation and waiting, the time was finally here. This was our first actual family vacation! Because we did not have the luxury of living near either of our parents, we had taken every opportunity we had to visit them. This meant we had to give up our own "family vacations." We were excited to be able to spend this time away together as a family.

The morning of our departure, a limousine came to our home to pick us up and take us to the airport. What service! The kids were amazed to be able to ride in this extra-special car! After a long weather delay and a short flight, we arrived in Orlando. Everyone was so excited to finally be on our way to Disney World. We were given the opportunity to stay at the Give Kids the World Village. We didn't get to the villa in enough time to go anywhere that first day, but we were able to look around the Village for a while. It was amazing in and of itself. There was so much for the kids to do, and because of the type of place that it is, we never had to worry about a cost associated with any of it. They even had an ice cream parlor open all day where we could enjoy all the ice cream we could eat—or at least all the ice cream that Daddy and Mommy would allow.

We enjoyed going to the different Disney parks and Sea World over the next five days, and we all had so much fun! It was great to watch the wonder and excitement in the kids' faces as we made our way through each park. As we toured the parks, we also enjoyed the many perks of being a "wish family." We didn't have to wait in lines, and Abby was treated well everywhere we went. One such highlight was Abby being the "captain" on the jungle safari river ride. She was even allowed to steer the boat. She felt pretty special and thoroughly enjoyed that opportunity. Emma got to experience her first ride on a "big roller coaster." Her excitement was contagious!

One of the favorites for the whole family was the fireworks

show. We all stood in awe at the impressive display of fireworks. I have to say that we also enjoyed the Sea World shows immensely as well. Overall, it was a big bundle of fun to be spoiled throughout that week. We were treated like royalty, and we thoroughly enjoyed our packed-full-of-activities trip. The week was a completely enjoyable time, full of wonderful memories for each of us. It was nice to enjoy the carefree vacation as a family!

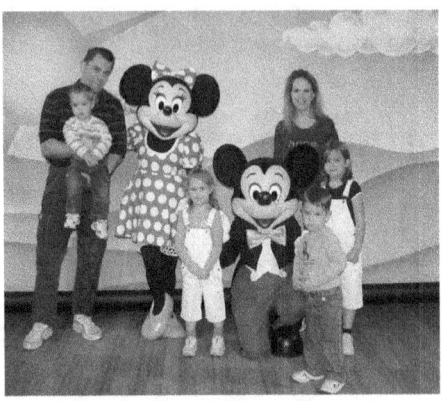

We were treated so well on our "Make a Wish" trip to Disney!

There are many Make-A-Wish families who are fulfilling their child's wish in hopes of some good final memories with their child. Thankfully, that wasn't the purpose of our trip. Abby was doing well; and for the time being, we didn't have to fear her cancer taking her life. We were able to enjoy it as a family vacation is intended to be.

We enjoyed this period of a few years that actually seemed normal. We felt as though we were pretty much like any other family; and life, in general, was going so well. We were definitely on a mountain top in our lives. We were thankful for the blessings that God had placed in our lives and for the lessons of faith and grace that He had given us.

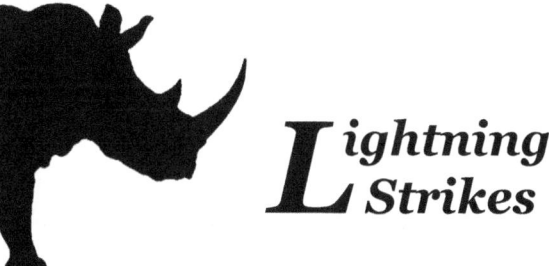

*L*ightning Strikes

Lightning Strikes

I have always enjoyed babies, especially *my* babies; and I loved that stage in my children's lives. To me, there was nothing more special than holding each of my babies for the first time. I loved meeting the child that I carried for so many months— to finally see what they looked like and be able to touch and hold them. I loved cuddling with them and talking "baby talk" to them. I loved singing their name to them. I loved seeing their "firsts," teaching them new things, and being the *one* that they want to have holding them. I loved being the one who could always get a smile out of them. Simply put, I have always loved the closeness and bonding that I experienced as a mother with my babies.

To our surprise, God decided that we weren't done having children, and we found out in May 2007 that we would be expecting our fifth child in January 2008. After the initial surprise, I quickly became excited about our new addition.

About a week later, we came back home from St. Jude where Abby had her last exam under anesthesia. We were excited because she was old enough now that she wouldn't need anesthesia for her eye exams. While I was there, I had told our friends at St. Jude that we were expecting again. For that matter, I had told our friends at home, too.

The day after I got home from Memphis, however, I started showing signs of an impending miscarriage. I went to the doctor, and he confirmed my fear that I was, in fact, going to lose the baby. Now how would I go back and tell everyone that I wasn't going to have a baby after all, without breaking down and revealing the deep pain in my heart?

The end of that month, I suffered a miscarriage, leaving me overwhelmed at the loss of the baby who had opened a new place in my heart. I was only six weeks pregnant when I lost that baby, but I was devastated because I had gotten to the point where I really *wanted* that baby. I had bonded with my baby for the previous two weeks, and I loved that baby so desperately. It came as such a shock to me to actually lose a baby because I had previously had four successful pregnancies. It never occurred to me that something would go this wrong.

I found myself often thinking about the child that I now would not be able to hold. I missed the idea of what that child would be. Was it a boy or girl? What would his personality have been like? How could I get over such a loss? I would never get to experience the joys of mothering that child, which left me deeply saddened.

I did, however, know that I would get to meet my precious baby someday in Heaven. This gave me much comfort as I thought about the loss I had sustained. I wouldn't get any further earthly joy from that child, but there would be eternal joy for the existence of a new soul in Heaven. I'm excited to think about the fact that Skip and I do have another child, and he or she is waiting for us.

King David spoke of his child that he had lost just seven days after birth and referred to seeing that child again. II Samuel 12:23 says, "But now he is dead, wherefore should I fast? Can I bring him back again? I shall go to him, but he shall not return to me." David said, "I shall go to him," which gave him comfort that they would see each other in Heaven some day.

Throughout the next weeks, I thought about and missed that sweet baby that I wouldn't know here on earth. At first, it was many times a day, and the tears would flow so easily. But after a while, the pain lessened. However, quite some time passed before I didn't think of that baby every day. I still experience some sadness as I think of my child.

Over the next couple of months, the Lord continued to heal my heart. After about five months or so, I decided that it would be best if we would be done adding to our family. I have since realized that, in reality, I really do not know what would be best. As I am writing the words, "*I decided* that it would be *best*," it now seems to be a very arrogant decision that I made seemingly in *my* best interest. No matter what we decide for ourselves, without the Lord's direction, we cannot be dogmatically certain that we are making the best choice for ourselves. We need to be sure that it is the Lord directing our steps and that we are seeking Him in making these decisions. He is the One who can clearly see the beginning from the end.

I was, however, content with the four beautiful children that God had given us, and I was ready to move on to the next stage in our lives since Zach was so close to being in school. The prospect of dropping all four children off at school seemed like a pleasant proposition. I would dream of all I could get done and enjoy while they were in school.

As I spoke to people after my miscarriage, I found out about so many women that I already knew who had lost a baby in the past. I was comforted by their stories of how the Lord brought healing in spite of their pain. I was able to share in their pain as they did in mine. It opened my eyes to a part of their lives that I hadn't seen before, and I was able to experience a much closer relationship with these women.

It also gave me opportunities to serve by comforting and having true empathy as I reached out to those who later found themselves experiencing similar heartache. Thankfully, God can use this seemingly-negative circumstance in my life. I am now able to help other women know of the hope and peace that can come even after such a great loss, telling them from first-hand experience how God helped me through it, and that He will do the same for them.

Skip had left the decision up to me whether or not we were "done" having children; he would be content either way. Yes, I had definitely decided I was ready to put the baby years behind me. Plus, I considered myself out of the "baby stage" because I could see and hold other babies and be able to not desire one of my own. Surely this would mean that we would end up being a family of six.

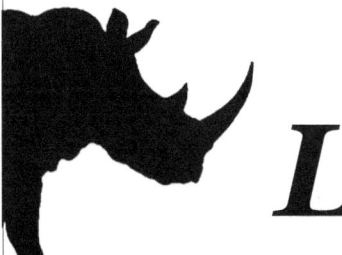

Losing A Parent

Losing A Parent

My dad had been battling renal cell carcinoma (cancer in the kidneys) since 2005, and in September 2007, he took a turn for the worse. I found myself making a couple of trips to Iowa to be with him and my mom. We didn't know how much time he had left, and his tumors weren't responding to any of the treatments anymore. He was running out of options.

When he was first diagnosed a couple of summers before, his cancer was in Stage IV. His long-term prognosis was not good. He had been on a few different treatments that worked for a while, only to find out that the effects weren't long-lasting. His disease would then continue to progress until another treatment was started, and the cancer would be held at bay a while longer.

The last two years had been rough, at times, and it was difficult to see the negative impact on my father and his body from the harsh treatments that he had to undergo. He was so sick and had so many side effects from the drugs. He had surgery to remove one of his kidneys and as much of the tumor possible; it ended up being the size of a football! He had lost so much weight, and it was so difficult to see him in such misery as he continued his treatments. I appreciated my visits with my father throughout this time, as I was forced to contemplate that one of these visits could be my last.

My time with him in October was good, and it was the last time I was able to spend any quality time with him. I enjoyed being with him and was thankful for the moments of humor that were so normal for his personality. These moments were somewhat scarce since he didn't feel well much of the time, but when that mischievous smile showed itself, it was absolutely wonderful.

Well, actually, those "moments of humor" may have better been described as "moments of embarrassment" for me as a teenager. Oh, what trying times I had as a teenager being the daughter of a man with such an extreme personality! As I grew up, I was able to laugh at his form of humor when I realized how much it didn't matter what others thought. Better yet, I realized that others didn't even think of me or my seeming plight with my father.

For example, and I don't think I'll forget this until the day I die, after one of his doctor appointments that October, we went out for lunch. The restaurant wasn't very full because we went at an odd time, but all of a sudden, I saw my dad wave at someone behind me. As I turned to see who it was, I saw a man swatting at a fly with his hand. He was eating alone, and I was relieved that he gave us a big grin as my dad waved at him, realizing that he saw the humor in my dad giving him a hard time about swatting at the fly. That was just something very typical of my dad. He wasn't shy in the least, and he really wasn't concerned about how others looked at him. He did love people, and in his own way, he tried his best to show it.

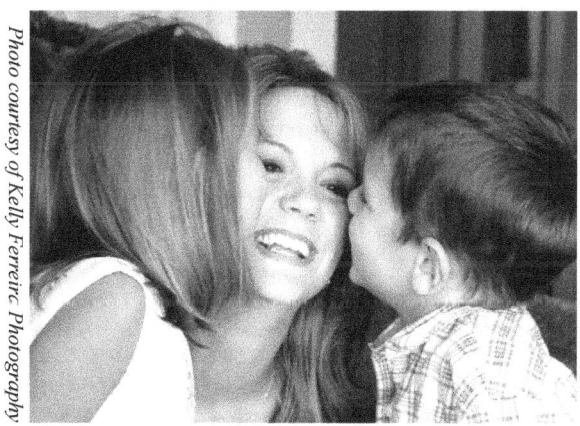

Photo courtesy of Kelly Ferreira Photography

I hope that Skip and I can pass on the faith and love my father gave me.

It was funny as I later thought about that occurrence; I would have been completely mortified as a teenager had my dad pulled something like that in public. I thought about the words that so often came out of my mouth: "Dad, stop it! You're embarrassing me!" Thankfully, since I've grown up, I've learned to appreciate his idiosyncrasies.

I have always said that the Lord used my dad to prepare me for my husband. I did as people often talk about—I married a man very similar to my father. Skip will often do and say so many things that I could see my dad doing or saying. It sometimes makes me think of fond memories of my dad, and sometimes it downright scares me! I was tremendously blessed in having these two wonderful men in my life!

My mom called me early in November and said that my dad was doing pretty poorly, and told me I should come up right away if I wanted to see him before he passed away. He wasn't awake or responsive anymore, and it was just a matter of time before his body would be forced to succumb to the cancer and its effects on his body. Skip and I decided that I should go immediately. He would stay with the kids and drive up when Dad had "gone home." I was able to spend the last couple days of his life with him in the hospital.

While I was there, I just wasn't able to bring myself to leave the hospital. I wanted to stay with my mom to help support her, and I didn't want to leave my dad. Because I felt I needed to be there for my mom when the time came, I spent the next two days and nights in the hospital with Dad and Mom, my sisters, and other relatives as they visited. I am very thankful we could be together for this difficult time. Early Sunday morning, November 11, 2007, I stood by my dad's bedside with my dear aunt (my dad's only sister) and my mother as he took his last breaths here on this earth. I consider it very appropriate that my dad went to Heaven on a Sunday morning, the Lord's day. In the past, my dad would always bring up the verse, Philippians 1:21, in which Paul says, "For to me to live is Christ, and to die is gain." Each time he quoted the verse, he would say, "I've never seen anything negative about gain, yet!" I knew he was ready to meet his Lord and Savior.

Upon learning that my dad had passed away, Skip started on the adventurous trip with four young children all by himself. Skip headed up to his parents in Indiana to spend the night, and then he drove over to Iowa the next day.

We had struggled with whether or not we wanted the kids,

or even maybe just the girls, to come over to Iowa for the funeral. With all that was going on, we decided that it would be best if Skip would just leave them there to spend time with their grandparents, aunt, and cousins, whom they didn't get to see very often. There were still plans and such that needed to be made that would be complicated by adding four children to the confusion. Plus, we weren't sure if they were ready for all that goes along with the funeral of a loved one. They were so young, and the trip would be difficult on them. It wasn't an easy decision, but we decided that it would be best for them to be able to spend the time with Skip's dad and mom in a happier environment. Skip came over to Iowa alone to be with me and my family.

As I reached out to the Lord, He again proved to be my comfort, reminding me that, as promised in the Bible, I would see my dad again in Heaven. I'm so thankful that I know my dad was a Christian; he had placed his trust in Jesus Christ. I remembered I Thessalonians 4:13, which says, we "*sorrow not, even as others which have no hope*" (emphasis mine) because we will be reunited one day. Later in that chapter in verse 18, we are instructed to "comfort one another with these words." The "others which have no hope" refers to those who are not saved. They don't have the hope of an eternity with Christ or an eternity with loved ones who have also gone to Heaven.

The wonderful thing is that this hope is available to everyone who wishes to receive it. All they need to do is to repent of their sins and put their faith and trust in Jesus Christ who gave His life for all. I have included a chapter at the end of this book that explains, through the Bible, how you can know for sure that you are ready and on your way to Heaven.

My dad's pain and suffering was finally at an end. He is much better off where he is, and compared to eternity, our separation will be just for a moment. God will always prove Himself faithful through the storms if we but reach for His hand!

It was difficult to think of the sadness to come as I would call their house in the future and not be able to hear his voice answer. Also, tears came to my eyes as I thought about not being able to enjoy his smile or laugh at his humor. But most of all, I was heartbroken for my mother who would now have to live without him.

Over the years since college, I had gotten used to not seeing my dad very often because I lived so far away. My life wouldn't be as dramatically impacted by his death, but her life would be so completely different. Her whole life had consisted of having my father there and focusing on his care. Now, she would be alone in the house with all of his things and memories. I hated the fact that she would now be so lonely. How would she fill her time? She did have the Lord, and I knew He would be her comfort throughout the months and years to follow.

Anyone who knew my dad knew that he loved to laugh and to make others laugh, but they also knew that he loved people and the Lord. His greatest desire was to love the Lord more each day than he had the day before. He was a wonderful father, and he gave me a great Christian heritage. I am so thankful that I know he was saved and will spend eternity in Heaven.

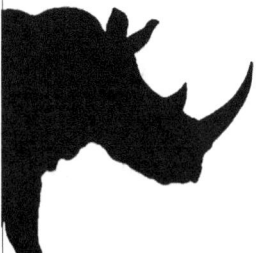

Robbing Peter to Pay Paul

*R*obbing Peter to Pay Paul

Throughout the next few months following my father's death, we went through a dark spiritual and physical storm—a *very* trying financial time. Winters in real estate tend to be pretty difficult financially because there aren't as many homes purchased throughout the winter season. Well, that winter proved to be no different.

Our real estate business in 2007 had slowed significantly. We sold substantially fewer homes that year, and it was making for a pretty dry winter without any savings stored up. We liken it to squirrels and ants. We need to gather as much as we can over the summer to make sure we have enough throughout the winter. To our dismay, there just wasn't anything extra that year to store.

The year 2006 had been very prosperous for us, bringing in a good income; yet we struggled the following winter. Another factor that added to our financial strain was that we also made the foolish assumption that since our income had increased each year for the previous three years, it would continue to do so. If nothing else, it would at least hold steady. Unfortunately, we were wrong.

We had previously made some unwise decisions, as well as some hasty decisions that had led to this financial valley. We had developed a way of life that required an income that was steadily good, instead of a conservative one that kept in mind the fluctuating real estate market. We hadn't planned for the future, and we certainly didn't plan for the downturn in the real estate market.

We had decided to purchase a new home on a snap decision before we sold our current home. We had also fallen for the extremely destructive lie that living on credit was "the American way of life." We had not heeded the red flags throughout the years that we were sinking deeper and deeper in credit card and consumer debt year after year. We justified our expenses that we put on credit by telling ourselves that it was *necessary*, without adjusting our budget and spending to live within our means. Well, actually, we foolishly didn't even live on a budget. It was too difficult to do on an income that fluctuated so much with the commissions earned, or so we told ourselves.

I do believe that God allows some trials in our lives as a consequence to sin. This was one of those trials. He can use these storms as well, with the hopeful outcome that we will change to be more like children after His own heart. The Old Testament is full of examples where the children of God would sin and be chastened. The trials and tribulations they went through had the desired effect. They would come back to the Lord for deliverance and draw themselves back into a right relationship with Him, experiencing blessing and prosperity in return.

God's goodness is evident. He cares enough to chastise us because He, the Creator, desires a close relationship with us. Psalm 94:12 says those who are chastened by God are blessed. Hebrews 12:6 and Revelation 3:19 tell us that God chastens us because He loves us!

We had now reached a time where we were feeling the consequences of the bad decisions we had made over the previous six years. We had not asked the Lord for His guidance before these hasty decisions that we had made, and we hadn't been good stewards of the funds that God had provided for our family. We now faced having to make payments with no money in the bank. Each month, we had four mortgage payments (a first and second mortgage on two different houses), a large SUV payment, credit cards, our other bills, and a second car payment—all of which we couldn't make when our income seemed to screech to a halt for the winter.

We had eventually gotten so low that we didn't even have money for a grocery run. We hadn't paid many of our bills for several months, and the stress mounted as the time passed with no present income and nothing coming in for the foreseeable future. Strangely, all of our real estate transactions during that time were for clients who chose to build their homes, and the closings were scheduled for months down the road after the homes were completed. We knew the time would be coming that we would have income, but what were we to do in the meantime?

The Lord wasn't opening any new doors, and any of the doors we tried to open for additional income, like finding other work or applying for jobs, were closed. We went through a time when we were praying and just waiting on the Lord for guidance, yet we weren't seeing the provisions He had showed in the past. He had always brought the right clients and timely closings to get us through.

At the lowest point of that emotional and physical valley, I had gotten to the point where I felt completely forsaken. In my mind, we couldn't get any lower financially. I wasn't angry or blaming God because I knew it was our own fault we were in this mess, but I did wonder why He wasn't providing as He had in previous circumstances. Why was it taking *so long* for the Lord to help or guide us? Throughout these five months of hardship, everything seemed to be crumbling all around us. How long could we go on like this?

Our financial crisis was proving to be a major stressor in our lives, and we were even beginning to feel the effects of the stress on our bodies. Our sleep patterns were being disturbed, and our normal body processes just weren't working as they should. It is amazing how your mental outlook can affect your physical being.

One night as I couldn't sleep, I got up and went into the bathroom to read my Bible, searching for any answer from the Lord. I don't normally think that opening the Bible and expecting an answer to be right there in front of my eyes is very effective, but I wasn't sure where to go. I was looking for some direction—any direction! I opened my Bible to Lamentations 3. I don't remember ever studying Lamentations or even reading much from it before. For some reason (obviously the Lord's leading), I opened my Bible to Lamentations 3. As I read the passage, I felt that the Lord was speaking directly to me regarding our exact circumstances! The first part of the chapter was as if it were coming from my heart and my mouth.

I read things like, "I am the man who hath seen affliction by the rod of his wrath." "Surely against me is he turned; he turneth his hand against me all the day." "He hath set me in dark places." "I cannot get out; he hath made my chain heavy." "Also when I cry and shout, he shutteth out my prayer." "He hath filled me with bitterness." "Thou hast removed my soul far off from peace; I forgot prosperity." "My strength and my hope is perished from the Lord." "My soul hath them still in remembrance, and is humbled in me." These were the *exact* things I was feeling in my heart. I was enraptured by the words as I read them.

But it also gave me hope as I continued reading the chapter. God revealed to me that He is compassionate and still faithful, even when we are in despair. I read in verses 21-36 things like, "This I recall to my mind; therefore have I hope." "It is of the Lord's mercies that we are not consumed, because his compassions fail not. They are new every morning; great is thy faithfulness." "The Lord is my portion...therefore will I hope in him." "The Lord is good unto them that wait for him, to the soul that seeketh him." "It is good that a man should both hope and quietly wait for the salvation of the Lord." "For the Lord will not cast off forever; but though he cause grief, yet will he have compassion according to the multitude of his mercies." "He doth not afflict willingly, nor grieve the children of men." Wow! There *was* hope!

The third part of the passage gave me instruction as to how to make my relationship right with the Lord. Verses 40-44 say, "Let us search and try our ways, and turn again to the Lord. Let us lift up our heart with our hands unto God in the heavens. We have transgressed and have rebelled; thou hast not pardoned. Thou has covered thyself with anger, and persecuted us; thou hast slain, thou hast not pitied. Thou hast covered thyself with a cloud, that our prayer should not pass through." Later the same passage reads, "Thou hast heard my voice." "Thou saidst, Fear not." "O Lord, thou hast pleaded the causes of my soul; thou hast redeemed my life." I knew then that I needed to let go, be patient, and trust the Lord. He would help provide the solutions to our financial problems.

That was an amazing spiritual experience! Reading that passage showed me that God is *real* in my life. He directed me to *that* passage, none other, and it was *exactly* what I needed to hear; it was the right passage at exactly the right time. I am so thankful for the comfort brought during this very difficult circumstance in our lives!

Every time I think about this passage and the hope it brought to me during one of my darkest spiritual times, it amazes me how the Lord just turned on the light, giving me comfort and relief. He was right by my side, even when I couldn't feel Him.

The valuable lessons that we have learned through that experience are ones that we will never forget. We have learned—and we hope we can help others to learn from our mistakes—that if your amount of debt increases from one year to the next, you *must* immediately take steps to reduce your debt! Never, never get to the point that the amount continually increases over time.

If you have found yourselves in a situation similar to ours, or if you feel you are headed in that direction, there are some financial institutions that are Christian-based that give wonderful financial advice and principles. (Information for contacting one example of these institutions can be found in the Resources section of this book.) We would encourage anyone to seek out this wise foundational help for your finances. Even if you are not in a dire circumstance regarding your finances, the principles that the Bible gives regarding finances are invaluable and are worth implementing in your budget.

This idea of readily-available credit is a horrible trap that so many Americans find themselves in! You can have the instant gratification of having the things you want, even when you don't have the money to pay for them. The idea is wonderful as far as temporary gain, but the price for it is harsh and lasting. There will eventually come a time when you realize that if you don't have the money for it now, you will not have it later when it comes time to "pay the piper." The better time to learn that is sooner, rather than later!

The world today often stresses through various media that instant gratification is what we should be able to expect. You shouldn't have to wait to have that item you want. The idea that you should save for the things you want is "old-fashioned," and that antiquated idea has no place in society today.

All of a sudden, you wake up and wonder how you ever allowed yourself to get to that point in the first place. You look back at all of the red flags that you should have seen but ignored. How foolish we can be in our finances. The negative effects far outweigh the temporary supposed "benefits" of spending on credit.

The prolonged financial state we had found ourselves in sealed in our minds that we *never* wanted to be in that position again, and we would make any necessary changes to avoid it in the future. We now have a very different philosophy on money and how we use it in our lives. We are still digging out of our debt, but we are no longer living on credit.

The difference between this storm and the storm with Abby a few years prior was that we knew there wasn't anything that we could do in our own strength to help Abby. We had to rely on the Lord to take care of her. This time, we knew that we should be doing whatever we could to fix the problem, but all of our feeble attempts proved to be futile. This actually made *this* storm darker in our lives.

It is difficult to admit these faults and air our "dirty laundry," but through our experiences with people, we have learned that many have found themselves in a similar position as ours. And, unfortunately, many others will have to learn the same lessons that we have. We are hoping and prayerful that our story of difficulty with finances will help others to avoid this situation, as well as encourage others who have found themselves in our shoes. We are not proud of where we found ourselves, but we pray the Lord can use our circumstances to help others in spite of ourselves.

We are actually thankful for that financial trial because of the invaluable lessons we learned. We often question why in the world we made those financial decisions, because now we see with clarity that a storm was the inevitable consequences of our actions. Unfortunately, it is only hindsight that is 20/20. We learned that you will reap *more* than you sow when making this kind of financial decision, and the results will be devastating.

Besides the financial lessons, one positive that resulted from this storm was the realization that even these tough times, that can so often drive a wedge in a marriage, can actually draw a couple closer. One key to having a positive outcome is to be sure not to play the "blame game." Skip and I both took equal responsibility, never blaming each other for our situation. We obviously could have, but that wouldn't have helped the situation. Thankfully Skip and I, by the grace of God, were able to stay close even during that stressful time. We knew we were in this together, and we would have to get out of it together. Having someone to rely on was so much better than having someone to blame.

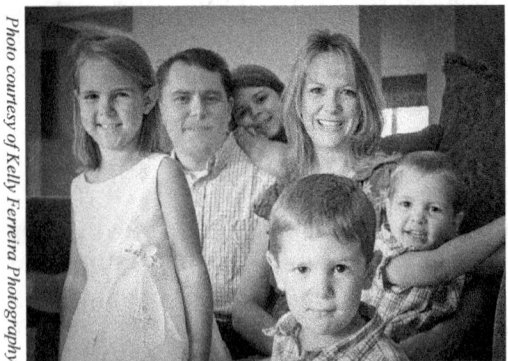

Even through the tough times, our family, faith, and relationships remained strong.

I need to continue to remember and implement the valuable lessons the Lord taught us through that time in our lives. When in the dark, I need to remember His goodness, grace, promises, and the light that He provided when I read the Bible that night. God often shows us a light to illuminate our current path, and that memory helps us in the future when we are in the dark again.

We will continue to have dark and light periods in our journey through the valleys and over the mountaintops of life. We just need to remember we are not alone when facing the darkness in the storms that we encounter.

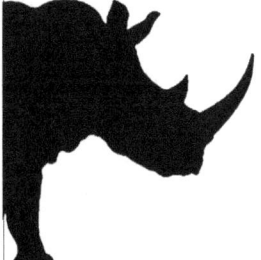

*L**earning From Job & Paul*

Learning From Job & Paul

I believe that God allowed all of these trials in our lives so that we could use the situations to point the glory back to God—in the same way that Job did. This was the story I heard over and over when God was preparing my heart—right before Abby's diagnosis of retinoblastoma. The story of Job showed me how important it is to trust God throughout a storm and to remain faithful—no matter how difficult times would get, and no matter what the storm.

The book of Job tells us the story of a man who had been blessed by God with great wealth, many children, and a wonderful life. The Bible describes him as "the greatest of all the men of the east" in Job 1:3. He followed God's laws and was a righteous man. His relationship with God was of utmost importance in his life. This relationship is the reason God said Job was righteous in His eyes. God did not consider Job to be righteous because he did not sin, but because he walked with God.

Because of Job's walk with God, God allowed Satan to test Job's faith. Satan stripped Job of all that he had. All of his children died; he lost all of his herds of animals. He lost it all. Though he lost everything, he still said, "The Lord gave, and the Lord hath taken away; blessed be the name of the Lord." The main point that we can apply to our lives is that, in spite of his great suffering, pain, and losses, he could still say, "Blessed be the name of the Lord." Job came into the world with nothing, and he acknowledged that he would leave with nothing, keeping his perspective focused on what is important.

But that wasn't all Job had to endure. Satan also afflicted him with physical ailments, consisting of terrible, painful boils completely covering his body. He was in extreme physical pain and suffered immensely with these boils, yet he remained faithful. He was under such dire circumstances that his wife told him to just "curse God, and die." To this he replied, "What? Shall we receive good at the hand of God, and shall we not receive evil?" He understood and acknowledged that all of the good he previously had in his life was from the Lord. He also knew it would be foolish to think that *only* good would come in his life without expecting any bad—he realized that storms are a part of life. Job was completely humbled, yet he still pointed to God's greatness. It seemed, from a human standpoint, that Job had nothing left to live for. Everyone in Job's life decided that because he was so severely afflicted, his suffering had to be a result of sin; yet Job maintained his righteousness and faithfulness.

Did Job despair over his circumstances? Yes—Chapter 3 tells us that Job wished he had never been born. Is it probable that we will go through trials without any lament for *our* situation? No, we are human; and to suffer is not what any of us wishes for our lives. Job grieved, but Job also remained righteous in God's eyes. The Bible gives him credit as a righteous and faithful child of God.

God doesn't expect us to go through storms with only a smile on our face, expressing joy at all times. God understands our grief, and He knows the feeling of intense suffering and heartache better than we do. He didn't condemn Job for grieving over his loss and pain. God is good; and while Job was suffering, God was with him through it all, providing the grace Job needed. Just like Job, all we need to do is remain faithful and trust God throughout the storm.

Paul gives us another perspective on how to remain faithful through storms and how we will ultimately be rewarded. We are told of all of the persecution and suffering that he endured for his faith and as a follower of Christ. Paul was mentioned in the Bible as a champion of faith. He was persecuted, stoned, beaten, imprisoned, and shipwrecked all during his ministry of preaching and teaching the Word of God. He went through many severe storms, yet he remained faithful to the work of the Lord. He kept his focus on God and kept doing what he knew was right.

Because of Paul's faith and walk with God, God was able to use him to pen a large portion of the New Testament to help teach others about living a life of faith. Paul made many references to suffering and eternal reward throughout the New Testament. In Romans 8:17-18, Paul says of Christians, "And if children, then heirs; heirs of God, and joint heirs with Christ; if so be that we suffer with him, that we may be also glorified together. For I reckon that the sufferings of this present time are not worthy to be compared with the glory which shall be revealed in us." He also says in II Timothy 2:3, 11-12, "Thou therefore, endure hardness, as a good soldier of Jesus Christ. It is a faithful saying: For if we be dead with him, we shall also live with him: If we suffer, we shall also reign with him: if we deny him, he also will deny us:"

Paul practiced what he preached; so much so, that ultimately he lost his physical life. He knew, however, that as he suffered through storms, there were still promises of God's faithfulness. Paul wrote in II Corinthians 4:7-9, "But we have this treasure in earthen vessels, that the excellency of the power may be of God, and not of us. We are troubled on every side, yet not distressed; we are perplexed, but not in despair; Persecuted, but not forsaken; cast down, but not destroyed."

Paul sums it up well in the verses of II Corinthians 12:9-10 when he says, "And he [speaking of Christ] said unto me, My grace is sufficient for thee, for my strength is made perfect in weakness." He goes on to confirm what that means in his life by saying, "Most gladly, therefore, will I rather glory in my infirmities, that the power of Christ may rest upon me. Therefore, I take pleasure in infirmities, in reproaches, in necessities, in persecutions, in distresses for Christ's sake; for when I am weak, then am I strong."

Along with Paul are many martyrs for the Christian faith who were persecuted and killed for their faithfulness to God. Paul's life was cut short, according to men's standards, but it was willingly given up for the cause of Christ and furthering His kingdom. Paul knew that his eternal reward would far outweigh his suffering here on earth.

It would be wise to consider that, very likely, our faithfulness and glorifying the Lord through our trials may not bring about earthly material benefits. We would be foolish to think that God would *owe* us anything in return for "our trouble."

We, on the other hand, owe God our love and loyalty because of His great provision of salvation. We need to keep in mind that God is worthy of all glory—not only because of who He is, but because of His provision for salvation, and because He has given us the grace to face the storms. An overview of Philippians 2:5-11 shows us Paul's attitude toward Jesus Christ and God. "Christ Jesus, who, being in the form of God...took upon him the form of a servant, and was made in the likeness of men; and being found in fashion as a man, he humbled himself and became obedient unto death, even the death of the cross. Wherefore, God also hath highly exalted him, and given him a name which is above every name, that at the name of Jesus every knee should bow, of things in heaven, and things in earth, and things under the earth, and that every tongue should confess that Jesus Christ is Lord, to the glory of God, the Father."

Paul will receive great reward in Heaven for his faithfulness and work for the Lord. Job and Paul were both mentioned in the Bible for their righteousness. Neither served God for any earthly compensation, but both will receive Heavenly compensation. This is ultimately the only compensation for faithfulness that should matter to any of us.

Every "thing" here on earth is of no value because the Bible tells us that the things of the world are temporary. "Things" are only worth wood, hay, and stubble and will be eventually destroyed; but the things of Heaven are forever. They are permanent; they will last for eternity. That should be the desire for our lives here on this earth—to serve God through our circumstances for a Heavenly reward.

Job is in Heaven today, according to the Bible, as a man of faith. While he did have the opportunity to enjoy restored earthly possessions before he died, I know that he would testify today of God's grace. It was worth keeping the faith through trials, even if he would have never reaped any earthly reward.

Our journey through the storms of having a child with

cancer, personal losses, or financial distress may not yield us any rewards here on this earth. However, our desire is to be faithful and to be a light and testimony through it all, pointing others to Christ so they also may benefit from the love and grace that is so readily available to help in times of need.

My hope is not that you will encounter storms, but that as you do encounter them, you can receive blessings comparable to those which we have experienced. The most effective way to thrive in a storm, as Job and Paul did, is by trusting God to see you through. He will provide the grace needed and reward your faithfulness. Little did we know that the lessons we had learned would be needed again in the near future.

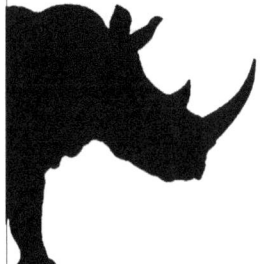

Blessing in Disguise

Blessing in Disguise

Through our entire financial storm, the Lord remained faithful and never let us go hungry. He provided for our needs by placing people in our lives that were a help to us. The blessings and lessons continued to come into our lives.

Right in the middle of that financial struggle, just after the New Year in 2008, we found out that we were very unexpectedly expecting! Well, it was clear that the Lord had other plans than my own family planning. There was no other explanation for my being pregnant. I wouldn't be done with just two girls and two boys after all. That really threw us for a loop! Why, when we are going through the worst financial time of our lives, would the Lord decide to give us a child? We were struggling to make ends meet, and here we find ourselves facing the need to provide for yet another child!

We found out the first Monday of the year that we were going to have another baby. It was the previous Friday that Skip and I watched a tow truck pull up to our SUV because we had fallen behind in our payments. Bewildered and in tears, I watched our truck get taken away. After that ordeal, you can imagine how the news of a new baby would add to the fear about our current financial state.

We decided that it would be foolish to try to get the truck back when we knew we would have a difficult time keeping up with the large payments. We would now need to look for a vehicle that we could purchase without a loan, and were very thankful when we found a good vehicle that would work for us. The only problem was that it seated six, and we would soon need a vehicle that could carry seven when the new baby arrived. But we knew that God would help us take care of that in His time; He was teaching us that *His* timing was not always going to match *our* timing.

At first, I had been hesitant to talk about my pregnancy because of the previous one that had ended in miscarriage. I didn't tell most people of our upcoming new arrival until I was 12 weeks along. I suppose there are a couple of reasons why I felt the need to wait to share the news. The first was partly because I feared the worst: a miscarriage. Secondly, the shame of the financial situation we had found ourselves in (though most didn't know the severity of it) caused me to be hesitant to share. I thought people would judge us and look down on us for making such a "poor decision" of having a child in spite of our circumstances. I didn't know how to explain that we tried hard *not* to get pregnant, and that this baby was the Lord's decision, not mine. I could hear the thoughts, "Yeah, right."

While I didn't desire anything but to have this baby, I felt guilty because I wasn't as excited about this pregnancy as I had been with my previous ones. I had already decided that I didn't want any more children, and we obviously weren't in a financial position to add a fifth child. I was also afraid to attach myself to this baby for fear that I would lose it. Again, God was teaching me that His ways are not my ways, and ready or not, a new bundle of joy was on its way.

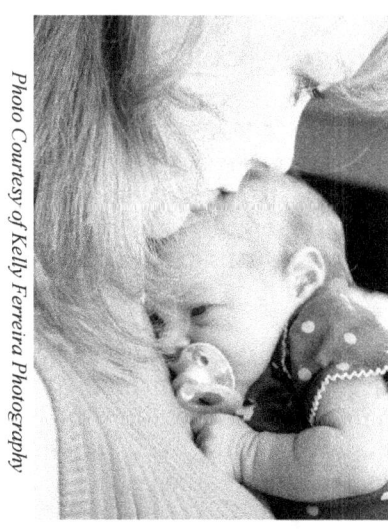

Looking back now at our precious child, we are thankful the Lord chose to give us this gift.

My ultrasound was coming up, which was a significant event for me during my pregnancies. I have always loved to see my babies on an ultrasound. I loved finding out if I was having a boy or a girl. (It was too difficult for me to wait to find out!) I wanted to know how to prepare for the arrival, and I wanted to be able to decide on and call my baby by name. I loved seeing the heartbeat and the movement to know that everything was all right. I loved to see the beautiful profile and tried to guess who the baby would look like. Most importantly, by this time, I had become excited about my new baby and being able to see him or her.

We brought all four of the other children to see their new brother or sister. The girls definitely hoped for a girl, and the boys were too young to care. Since my previous pregnancy, I had often thought about how much I would like for my "baby" to be a girl, mostly because I love the relationship I have with my mother. In my mind, there is nothing like a friendship and relationship of a mother and daughter. I thought about how wonderful it would be to have another girl and to be able to dress her up in all of the pretty little-girl things. Even though I truly would have been happy with either a boy or girl, I was elated when the technician told me that I was having a girl.

After the ultrasound was finished, the technician told me to wait in one of the exam rooms, and that my doctor would see me in a few minutes. As I waited for her, I reveled in my excitement about another baby girl. The doctor came in, and told me that there were a couple of things on the ultrasound that caused concern. This is every mother's fear—that something may be wrong with her baby.

My doctor said that the baby had a "short nasal bone," and the pictures showed she had a club foot. She said that either of these alone wouldn't be too much cause for concern. Since there were both issues, however, she was concerned that my baby girl had Down syndrome. Because of this, she referred me to a Maternal-Fetal specialist for a follow-up ultrasound. I made an appointment for a couple of weeks down the road, and all I could do was wonder about the health of this baby.

Hearing that my baby could have Down syndrome came as a surprise, but I knew that this baby was given to me by the Lord and there was no mistake. I was mostly concerned for my baby girl about what a difficult life she would lead. I was saddened that she might have to deal with so many struggles.

I began to research Down syndrome and checked into local support groups for families who have children with Down syndrome. I read over and over about how loving these children are and what a joy they are to their families in spite of their disabilities. My research also made me realize that most likely this baby would never be independent. Skip and I would have to take care of her for her entire life. Many who know Skip have probably heard him tell his philosophy on having children—I can have as many children as I want, but at a certain point, we would need to be done. Not only that, but we need to have them quickly—"get 'em in, get 'em out." He didn't want to raise children in our "old age," and he wanted to be able to retire without kids so we could travel. In his words, "It's hard to have a motor home with a bumper sticker that says 'If you see my kids, don't tell them you saw me 'cause I'm spending their inheritance' with kids hanging out the windows." Having a child in our home for the rest of her life wasn't exactly what we had planned.

I have a friend who has a baby with Down syndrome who is so sweet and lovable. God has done a work in their family because of His gift of this child. While it gives them challenges, she is still a blessing to the family. I knew I could look to them for encouragement and help with raising a special-needs child.

I also thought about the possibility that maybe she *didn't* have Down syndrome. After all, my doctor only suspected that she had this disability. As I thought about this scenario, I realized that she would still have a tough road ahead because of her club foot. She would need to have surgery to fix it, even if she didn't have to face the delays of Down syndrome. Either way would be difficult—delays and surgery, or just surgery.

You can imagine the thoughts that ran through my mind those next two or so weeks while I waited for my ultrasound with the perinatologist. I had mixed feelings, happy and sad. After all, a mother's primary hope during pregnancy is generally that the baby is healthy. I could think of the blessings she would bring, as well as the difficulties that our whole family would face as a result of a special-needs child. We were no stranger to this concept.

We went in for our ultrasound and watched the amazing pictures of our beautiful baby. After looking for the concerns that my technician and doctor had brought up, they told us that she *didn't* have a club foot. They said that she did have a short nasal bone, but that it wasn't much of a concern. They said I could have an amniocentesis to make sure that she didn't have Down syndrome, but I knew that it wouldn't matter either way. I opted not to have the amino testing done.

Praise the Lord! She didn't have a club foot. That possibility was ruled out, and therefore made the possibility of Down syndrome much lower. Looking at her profile during that ultrasound, we could see a huge similarity to Zach's profile. The nasal bone and profile looked just like his. The "short nasal bone" seems to be a trait that all of our children have. We were pretty much relieved of our fears, but the doctor wanted to follow up in a few weeks to be sure. I could now dream about my perfectly healthy baby girl.

We went in for the follow-up visit to the perinatologist for yet another ultrasound. I didn't mind because I loved seeing the ultrasounds of my developing baby. The doctor confirmed that the previous concerns would be pretty much alleviated. There was no club foot, and the nasal bone was fine. There was very little fear of her having Down syndrome at this point, but now he brought up a new concern. He said that one of the baby's kidneys was considerably smaller than the other one, and that there were "spots" on one of them. He said he wasn't largely concerned because there was enough amniotic fluid for us to believe there was enough output from the kidneys. He also said it might resolve itself because these things often do, but he wanted to check on her in a few more weeks.

I began to research the concerns of the cysts on her kidneys, but I didn't allow myself to dwell on it much since the doctor didn't make a big deal out of it. It could have been a problem in that she would only have one functioning kidney and be totally reliant on the one. However, there was too much else going on in my life, which I will cover in the next chapter, to decide to worry about the unknown. God was going to have to take care of the details. I knew He would help me through whatever it would take to care for my new baby.

This was a personal emotional storm; I was an expectant mother concerned about the health of my unborn baby. I am thankful for the moments I could spend contemplating God's purpose for each child He places into our lives. Again, I was able to realize that God did not make a mistake in giving my baby life at this time. You always hear mothers say that as long as the child is healthy, that is all that matters. Well, sometimes we have to realize that blessings also come in the form of a child that we may not consider "healthy," and even sometimes during a time that we may not consider convenient.

Sure enough, when we went in for the repeat follow-up ultrasound, the baby's kidneys looked just fine. She looked like a perfect, healthy baby girl! We had gone from this roller coaster of fears and concerns for our new baby girl, to having a feeling that we would have a healthy child. Still, God was teaching us, yet again, to trust in Him. And we would.

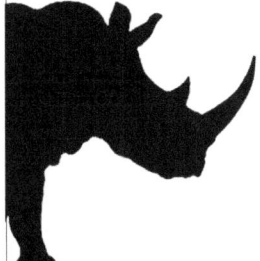# A Time for Rejoicing

A Time for Rejoicing

May 2008 came about with the *normal* things in our life... real estate started to pick up for the summer, helping to put an end to our financial crisis, the kids finished up the school year, and I continued my job as Mommy, wife, and real estate assistant.

Abby turned six that month, and we were feeling pretty good about her overall health. She had just been to her checkup at St. Jude the month before, and everything looked great. That appointment in April was also the appointment where she "graduated" to the next level—to their ACT (After Completion of Therapy) clinic. She would not need medical care, and she now would just receive follow-up and research care. She had continued to do very well with the retinoblastoma, and she had still been able to keep both of her eyes. We were more than pleased with the status of her health, considering her rough start to life!

Throughout pretty much the entire month of May, however, Abby had been limping without any explanation. She limped for so long that I thought she was just limping out of habit—or maybe for attention. I told her a few times to "walk right." She would try, but she would go back to limping. When we first noticed the limp, we couldn't think of anything that she had done to hurt her leg. When we asked her, she didn't know of anything that she had done to hurt it either. Maybe it was just growing pains—it didn't seem to hurt her too badly; it was more of a nagging pain.

After about three weeks, the pain got worse—to the point that if she stepped wrong, she would cry out in pain. At this point, Skip and I decided to take her to the doctor. It was obvious then that she wasn't limping for attention or out of habit, and it was worse than growing pains. They did an x-ray which showed nothing. Because of her medical history, however, the doctor wasn't satisfied with not finding the source of the pain; he ordered an MRI.

Little did we know that this was the start of an emotional roller coaster through which the Lord would continue to strengthen our faith. Abby's MRI was scheduled on a Saturday, so we knew we probably wouldn't get the results until Monday. The radiologist would need time to read it and get the results to the pediatrician. Monday came and went, and we were feeling pretty good about the results. We were sure we would have been contacted right away if anything suspicious showed up. In our previous experience, we'd found that the doctors give immediate attention to something that is potentially serious.

Tuesday came around, and we were still waiting for the results. At the end of the day, we finally got a call from the doctor who told us that the MRI did show an abnormality in her left leg just above the knee. He contacted the doctors at St. Jude who obviously wanted to see her right away. In fact, Abby's oncologist from St. Jude even called me personally a few minutes later about bringing Abby up to Memphis to be checked out.

I remember going to the monthly ladies meeting at our church that night after hearing about Abby's MRI results. Some of the ladies cried with me at the thought of something being wrong with Abby. We were afraid that Abby and our family would be going through more cancer treatments. I also remember meeting a lady that night who didn't go to our church, but she came as a visitor to our ladies meeting. She told me that she had lost her daughter at the age of six, I believe, to cancer. I was hoping that I wasn't being prepared for the worst news.

I picked up the MRI results to take to Memphis and looked at the report. It said that there was an "abnormality in the bone marrow, extending into the surrounding tissue." This was very scary to read because, in my mind, that could only mean one thing—cancer was present. What else could cause a report like this?

Just a few days after we received Abby's MRI results, my mom, who just happened to be visiting me at the time, and I took Abby to St. Jude for further tests. Skip decided that he needed to stay home to work on improving our financial situation.

While we were there, they did a bone scan and another x-ray. Her oncologist told us that all of the signs were not good—that they pointed to osteosarcoma, a cancerous tumor in the bone. It presented just as osteosarcoma would. It was in the right place; it caused her pain; and she was at a high risk because of her history.

She was, however, *very young* to have osteosarcoma; it usually doesn't affect children younger than ten years of age. Abby was barely six. Actually, she was still five when she started limping. Also, the pain in her leg had subsided dramatically, and she no longer was walking with a limp. She would walk, run, and jump like usual. This was a good sign that it was healing. If it were cancer, the fear was that the pain would get progressively worse, not better. Her doctor seemed to think that if it *was* cancer, the pain would be bad enough to wake her up at night, and it hadn't been.

Her doctor got the test results the next day, and he told us that it looked like the problem with her leg was only a stress fracture. He told us he wanted to follow up with her in six weeks to make sure that was the case, and that it was healing properly. I called Skip to tell him the wonderful news—Abby just had a stress fracture. Well, at the time that I called him, Skip was on the side of the road changing a flat tire under some not-so-pleasant circumstances. However, his difficulties all diminished when he realized how thankful he was for "just a broken leg"! As he told me about this later, I couldn't help but laugh. It was so cute how even in his current difficulty, changing the flat tire, he was absolutely elated and didn't care about anything else when he heard the words "she just has a stress fracture." He praised the Lord for "a broken leg" throughout the day.

We came home in the next day or so and resumed our life as usual—glad to put that behind us. I'm sure you can imagine our relief after the intense concern we had about Abby's leg. Life was good again, back to normal.

I planned a trip to Iowa in July to surprise my mom for her 60th birthday. Because it was her first birthday without my dad, I wanted to be there for her. It worked out pretty well

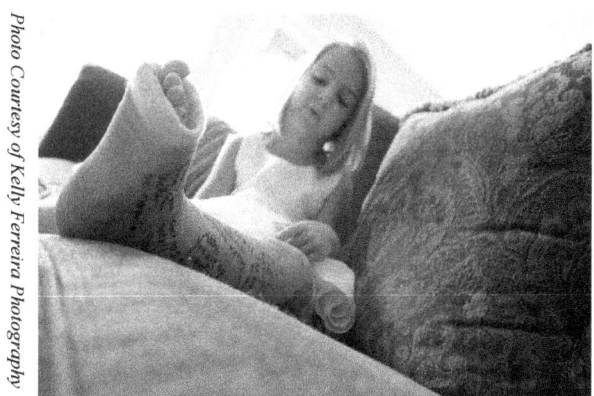

Abby with her bright pink cast and lots of supporters

since Mom's birthday was just a few days before Abby's next appointment (which, actually, was on my dad's birthday). We could just stop in Memphis, since it was right on our way home.

My last follow-up ultrasound was scheduled early in the second week of July. Because I planned to leave from there to head to Iowa, Skip and the kids went with me for my ultrasound, with everything packed and ready to leave afterwards. This was the ultrasound where we found out that the baby's kidneys were normal and there were no further health concerns with her.

Because of his real estate schedule, Skip wasn't able to go to Iowa with me. Apparently, sanity has never really been my strong suit. Looking back, it seems a little crazy for a pregnant woman, in her last trimester, to travel *that far* with four children—a just-turned eight-year-old down to a barely-three-year-old—with no help. So seven months pregnant, I packed up the four kids for my ten-hour drive to Indiana for an overnight stop at Skip's parents, and then another ten hours on to Iowa. Though it seemed crazy, I took the trip, knowing that taking all four children was my only option. Thankfully, the trip was uneventful.

We arrived safely in Iowa, and the surprise was successful. The kids reveled in the fact that Grandma was surprised—we had pulled it off! We had a big birthday party that weekend where I was able to see so many people I hadn't seen in several years. They were able to meet my kids, and we had a great time with family and friends. We spent a few days in Iowa, but it was all-too-soon time to leave.

After our pleasant visit, the kids and I headed down to Memphis for Abby's follow-up appointments. It was difficult to leave. I was disappointed that I couldn't spend the next day, my dad's birthday, with my mom. I knew it would be a difficult day for her. The plan was to spend a couple of days at St. Jude for Abby's appointments and then head back to our normal lives at home in Florida for some much-needed rest for me. This proved to be just the midpoint of our emotional roller coaster.

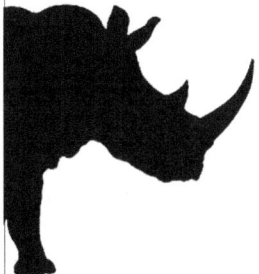

The Unexpected News

The Unexpected News

That week, we would again learn how the Lord helps us to see in the dark. We went to St. Jude Children's Research Hospital on Wednesday morning for Abby's scheduled appointments. After a new x-ray and other tests, we met with Abby's oncologist. He confirmed our initial fear: the new x-rays showed bone deterioration, causing him to believe that Abby did, in fact, have osteosarcoma. They would need to do a biopsy for an official diagnosis; that was scheduled for that Friday.

This time, I was by myself when I heard the news; well, by myself with four children and the doctor. Thankfully, I knew I needed to keep my reaction low-key. The children were enough of a distraction, so I received the news fairly well. Also, because of our previous concern a few weeks earlier, it didn't necessarily come as a surprise. The Lord was with me and gave me the comfort I needed. *Cancer, Wow!*—here we go again.

Now I would have to call Skip and tell him the dreaded news. *This* phone call wasn't nearly as easy or pleasant as the one after our last visit with her doctor in Memphis. I didn't have a message of relief to deliver this time.

Our present circumstances sent our minds into a whirlwind of what to do. How would we make this work? Skip had already stayed home from our trip to Iowa because of business. How would we work out what needed to be done over the next few days? Skip knew he now needed to make the trip to Memphis somehow. He would have to tie up as much as he could with the real estate business and head our way.

Throughout the next couple of days, they did further testing, and we agreed on a treatment plan for Abby. They needed to do a chest CT to check for metastasis to her lungs, since that is the next place for osteosarcoma to spread. Thankfully, her lungs were clear, and we wouldn't have to face additional treatment associated with that. Because it usually doesn't take long for this aggressive disease to go to the lungs, we were thankful that we caught it before this happened.

The protocol she would be on included eight months of chemotherapy and major surgery to remove the tumor in her leg, including the affected part of the femur as well as possibly the knee joint. This would mean a *nine-month stay* in Memphis. We had so many decisions to make at this point.

Skip and I decided he would come up for her biopsy, stay a few days, and take Emma, Micah, and Zach home early the next week. I would stay in Memphis with Abby. Because of the schedule of treatments, Abby and I would have to *live* in Memphis throughout her treatment—making the situation much more difficult. We now faced the grim prospect of our family being separated for a very long period of time.

Skip and I have always been a very close couple. We don't usually spend very much time apart. At most, maybe a week or so while I took the kids to visit my family or Skip's family. Even then, we hated being separated for that long. We spent the previous years working and doing pretty much everything together, 24 hours a day. We didn't even have separate hobbies. We were teased by some that we were "attached at the hip." Well, now we would both have to function as single parents for several months.

On top of all of these circumstances—Abby's new fight and the separation of our family—we had to try to figure out what to do about the new addition that would join us in less than *two months*. I was at the point where I would be seeing my doctor every two weeks, and soon thereafter, every week. How and where would I be able to have this baby, now that I would be living in Memphis? I didn't have a doctor in Memphis, and how would I even be able to find one at this stage in my pregnancy? Plus, I still had to take care of Abby and her needs. At what point would this fifth baby decide to come? What if she would be weeks early?

You know, through this time, I again began to wonder why the Lord decided to give us a baby *now*. I just could not understand—it was beyond me! We definitely hadn't planned this baby who would be joining us very soon. We knew the Lord would work out the details. For the time being, we needed to focus on Abby and helping her get started along this new journey we unexpectedly found ourselves on.

Her doctor told us before the surgery that they would be able to tell during the biopsy whether it was, indeed, osteosarcoma (even though everyone was already sure of the diagnosis). If the tissue they saw confirmed their suspicions, they would go ahead and perform an additional surgery, while she was already under the anesthesia, to insert a subcutaneous port in her chest. They would use it to administer her chemo, have direct access to her veins for blood draws, and give her the other intravenous medications she would need. When she came out of surgery with a port, it sealed in our minds what we were facing. They would still send the tissue sample for accurate diagnosis, but everyone already knew what we were up against. We were going to go ahead with her previously-planned treatment protocol.

After Abby's biopsy that Friday, they put a cast on her leg from her toes to just above the middle of her thigh and gave her a set of crutches. They also gave her a wheelchair to use while she was healing from the biopsy. For the first couple of weeks after the surgery, even the slightest movement caused an immense amount of pain—poor thing! Because of the extreme pain, she used the wheelchair pretty much full-time for a few weeks.

We were, once again, staying with some of my family (distant relatives) who live in the area. We were so blessed by having them there in the Memphis area throughout the years of Abby being treated at St. Jude. We first met Scot and Jill when Abby was diagnosed in 2002, and they have been such a blessing to our family ever since.

Because St. Jude can allow only four family members to stay overnight in any of their provided housing, having a family of any more than four poses a problem—where to stay? Scot and Jill were always available to either keep the "extra" kids or even allow the whole family to stay with them. This helped us avoid the cost and hassle of having to get a hotel room, and it gave us a much more comfortable place to stay. We were so thankful to be able to stay with them while we were all in Memphis.

The first night after Abby's biopsy, in spite of the pain medications, she would scream out in pain even at the slightest movement of her leg. We were beside ourselves to know how to help her. She was at her maximum dose of pain meds, but they didn't seem to even touch her pain. All we could do was get her as comfortable as possible so she wouldn't need to move. We propped her up with pillows and made her as comfortable as we could just to get her through the night.

The two or three days after Abby's biopsy, the severe pain in her leg continued. As her mother, it was so difficult to see her like that, and it was difficult to know what to do for her since the pain medicine wasn't helping as much as we would have liked. Thankfully, as they adjusted her pain medications, her pain was better controlled over the next few days.

Skip, along with Emma, Micah, and Zach, left early the next week. It was so hard to say goodbye to my "Florida four," not knowing how frequent our visits would be. My poor children, especially Emma, who was old enough to understand—had to leave knowing I wouldn't be coming home for quite some time.

As if the heartache of leaving Abby behind in her state wasn't enough, Skip had a tremendously rough trip home that day. As I mentioned earlier, during our trip to Memphis in June, Skip had been by the side of the road changing a flat tire when I called. On this trip, he realized that it wasn't an isolated problem with the "new" tires that were on the car when we purchased it. On his 450-mile trip home, all three of the other tires went bad (!!!), causing many delays and headaches for my poor, already-bewildered husband. Late into the night, he safely arrived home after his extremely prolonged and bumpy ride.

Then reality began to set in; I would be caring for Abby by myself. I would be the one that the bulk of the responsibility would fall on to care for her. Even being 7-1/2 months along in my pregnancy, with my hormones swelling, I had to be strong for Abby's sake. I realized none of this could be about me.

Abby handled the diagnosis and news of her treatment amazingly well. She didn't remember anything she had been through as a baby and young child. To her, cancer wasn't that scary. She knew that she already had cancer, but she didn't remember any of the ill effects of it. There was very little fear associated with learning of her new disease.

We also needed to decide what we would do for Abby's schooling. She had attended 4-year-old kindergarten and 5-year-old kindergarten at a private school in our area, and she had done very well academically. We needed to basically decide whether she would attend school at St. Jude, or whether I would homeschool her, since we were going to be living in Memphis for the school year. We decided the easiest thing in our situation would be for her to attend school there at the hospital. They had developed a system that worked for the special situation these kids are in, and she would go to school three days a week from 11 a.m. to noon.

We realized early on that this was a *whole different battle* than Abby's first cancer, and we would be dealing with more invasive procedures and stronger chemo. When she was a baby, we would fly in, get her chemo, and pretty much just fly back home. Now, we would have to live, eat, drink, and breathe cancer treatments—this would be a permanent part of our immediate future. That just meant to us, however, that the grace of God would be that much stronger in our lives this time around. God promises us that He will not give us more than we can handle, and we were clinging to this promise.

While it was difficult for Skip and me to learn of Abby's newly-discovered diagnosis, we knew we were helped through a similar situation before. We liken it to standing in a lit room, preparing to turn out the light. You look at your route and memorize it, so after you turn out the light, you can still "see" your path in the dark. We were so thankful to be able to see in the darkness what the Lord had shown us in the light, and we were confident that He would remain by our side through this journey as well. We've used this "seeing in the dark what we saw in the light" many times throughout the past few years as we've gone through storms.

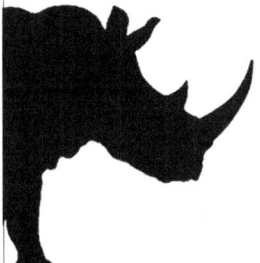

Another Go-Around

Another Go-Around

As Skip, Emma, Micah, and Zach left at the beginning of the next week, Abby and I stayed to begin her treatments. This was *not* supposed to happen! I was supposed to be going *home* from Memphis as I was traveling back from Iowa. I wasn't prepared to live in Memphis! I didn't have the things I would need from home to actually live there; I only had the things I would normally take to travel on a one-week trip. I was reminded that there is a wonderful security in a family being able to function together as a unit.

I longed for nothing but to be going home with Skip and all the kids—and just to be our normal family. But that wasn't the case, no matter what I longed for. Here we had gone from fear of cancer, to relief of no cancer, to the grim truth that the cancer was, in fact, a reality. Our lives were now completely upside-down again!

That week Abby started her first round of chemotherapy, and all of its terrible side effects kicked in. The first round consisted of two drugs—cisplatin (which is the cousin drug to the carboplatin I referred to that she had as a baby, which can cause hearing loss) followed by doxorubicin (cis/dox combo). Cisplatin is such a harsh drug, and it took its toll on her body with a vengeance! Abby was so *terribly* sick! She vomited over and over even after there wasn't anything left. Her leg was still in extreme pain whenever she moved. How would we make it through so many months of this? As her mother, it was extremely difficult to know there was so very little I could do to make it better for her.

My sweet, little Abby was so pitiful. It was seldom that there was a smile on her face. Every once in a while, something would amuse her or please her enough that she would muster one. Oh how I relished each of those rare smiles! Please understand, Abby was the child who would often get in trouble for being too silly. She always giggled and laughed, and she found humor in everything! She was an absolutely happy girl before this.

She would take things too far, and I can remember, after she was scolded for it, seeing her try to hide her smile from me because she just couldn't help it. Now, though, she was so out of character. It was so sad to not see that beautiful smile; she just didn't feel good.

Thankfully, the doctors know how to help these children with their sickness, and the medications allowed her to be sedated for much of the time. This was in hopes that she would sleep through a lot of her recovery and stay relaxed enough to feel okay when she was awake. She was given steroids and three different medications just to try to keep her nausea under control. She was on fairly strong pain medication for her leg as well. There is a learning curve, at first, for them to figure out what will work for each individual child and to determine what mix of medications will help them most effectively. That first round of such a harsh chemo drug really took its toll on her little body, and they were learning what she would need in order to be as comfortable as possible. Because of her sedation, Abby didn't remember much about her hospital stay for that first round of chemo. It was a blessing that she wouldn't have to remember the miserable condition she endured.

As her mother, watching Abby go through such distress was difficult. Adding to that, a nurse came into Abby's hospital room one day to teach me how to give Abby her shots. There is a drug that counters the effects of the chemo and helps bring the blood counts up faster after chemo administration. Unfortunately, it came in the form of a shot, which I had to give her in her leg. They gave me no choice; I had to do it. I knew it was best for Abby, but that didn't make it any easier for me to give it to her. So, here is my baby girl feeling absolutely horrible from the chemo, her leg is so sore she can't move it, and now I am forced to inflict more pain on her.

It absolutely crushed me, and tears streamed down my face as I gave her that first shot! All I could do, as she looked into my eyes crying, was say, "I'm sorry, *I'm sorry!*" It was awful seeing the look in her eyes. It was as if she didn't understand why I was hurting her. I felt like the worst mother, but I knew I was doing it for her own good. I realized it is extremely difficult to play nurse *and* mother.

Well, the shots had to continue daily until her counts rebounded, but the Lord gave us the grace, and we made it through them. She really was very brave. In fact, throughout the last several years, when she needed to have blood drawn from her arm for lab work, and she wouldn't even whimper or flinch. She would just put her arm out, let them take the blood, and it was done without a fuss or even a single tear. I was so proud of her!

Abby's doctor and I tried to explain things to Abby about what was happening and what was going to happen. She seemed to take it all pretty well until we told her that her hair would fall out. She started to cry, but it was fairly short-lived. She was actually pretty weepy because of the medicine, so I wasn't sure how she would handle it when the time came. Ultimately, because of her sedation and other medications, Abby didn't even remember that conversation.

During her hospital stay for the first round of chemo, St. Jude had finalized our housing. Because of our long-term stay, we would be housed in the Target House, consisting of two-bedroom apartments for the families, at no cost, during treatment. My mom and I moved into the apartment that week, and when Abby got out of the hospital, we were able to take her to her new "home."

The Target House was a huge blessing to our family throughout our stay in Memphis. It was a perfect blend of home and distractions for the families. There were many different things for the kids to do there, but Abby was so sick and in pain the first few weeks that we weren't able to fully enjoy the amenities.

After that first round of chemo, Abby had a couple of weeks off before her next round. As soon as her blood counts rebounded, they said we could go home for a few days. This was a relief because I still wanted to get some of my things from home, and I needed to see my obstetrician so we could "plan" the birth of our new arrival in a month or so.

One problem that came along with my not being home, was trying to work out how Skip could do everything by himself. He had three children to take care of (two of them would be starting school soon and getting out of school at different times), taking care of the house, laundry, making meals, and much more. This was all in addition to working the real estate business alone to be able to support the family.

In the past, we had been working our real estate business together. I had done pretty much all of the computer work, contracts, files, e-mails, and more. Now he was going to have to do pretty much all of it *alone,* not to mention suddenly becoming a single dad with all of those responsibilities! He had such a tough role in all of this, and he handled it all amazingly well with the Lord's help.

Many people were graciously able to help out so much here and there. Our church family rallied around us and did whatever they could to help us. They were there to provide meals, childcare, and help clean. The blessings that we received through others, who allowed the Lord to work through them, are ones that we will not soon forget!

Abby's counts finally came back up enough for us to be able to come home for a visit, and we were so thankful to be reunited with our family. It was strange, though, to be visiting our home. I felt I was in a completely different role while I was home—almost like I was visiting Skip's house. It was an odd feeling, but I didn't feel like it was *my* home. Skip and I do things differently, and I needed to adjust to how things were while I was gone. It was a little disconcerting to feel that way while I was home, but that was where we had found ourselves. We needed to learn to deal with it for the time being.

Also, Abby now had to get around the house with a cast and crutches. They initially decided to place the cast on Abby's leg, which went from her toes to a little above the middle of her thigh, with the thought that she would get it off when the fracture and biopsy site healed. Because of her cast, she now had to deal with itching, awkwardness, and difficulty keeping up with Emma, Micah, and Zach.

While we were home on that visit, we were able to get some family pictures with my friend Kelly, who is a wonderful photographer. We were so thankful for that opportunity, as it was just days before Abby completely lost her hair. It was wonderful to see her happy again after the effects of her chemo had mostly worn off. We enjoyed a little bit of "normal" for a few days.

Abby's hair began to fall out pretty quickly after that. Every day, handfuls were gone. Abby took it in stride, and she never complained about it one bit. She knew it was part of the treatment, and since there wasn't anything that could be done about it, she didn't even bother fighting it. I think it helped that she had seen so many children at St. Jude without hair, so it didn't feel so distressing. When most of it had fallen out, I asked her if she would like for me to cut the last few strands off. She said yes, and from then on she got used to having no hair. She didn't let any of the stares bother her, and for the most part, people were very understanding and gracious to her.

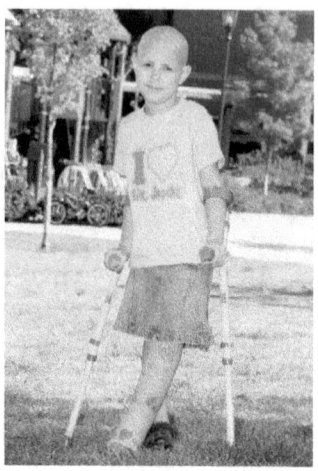

Abby at the Target House in Memphis

I was able to make an appointment with my obstetrician. We knew this would be the last one before the birth because there weren't any more breaks in Abby's schedule for us to come home. I met with my doctor, and she said everything looked good with the baby and me. We made plans that I would come home and be induced early in September. Because of the circumstances, we decided it would be best to plan the birth two weeks early, instead of being surprised by the baby possibly coming early in Memphis. This way, we felt it would be pretty safe that I would be able to have the baby back home, and it was almost certain that Skip would be able to be present for the birth. We also were trying to fit our new baby's birth into Abby's chemo schedule. I hoped to be able to spend about three weeks at home before having to go back to Memphis.

Abby was able to attend Vacation Bible School at our church that week; she was so excited that we were home for that. During this week, she began to learn of her limitations; as the other children played games and did activities that she couldn't do, she often had to sit on the sidelines and watch them play. She did very well with her lessons, however, and won a Bible for her hard work that week. She was so pleased with her new Bible.

During this visit home, I was also able to assess what I needed to take back with me for my extended stay. I was thankful for this opportunity, and I felt more prepared. Unfortunately, it was already time to head back to Memphis for Abby's next round of chemo. The separation was very difficult on each one of us. How I longed for the security of being able to stay home together as a family.

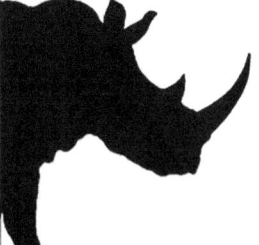

Preparing for the New Addition

Preparing for the New Addition

I am continually amazed at what the Lord brought us through. As I recall the details of our lives during this journey, I wonder how we would ever have been able to weather this storm without the Lord! Because the Lord gave us Abby, and He also gave us the new baby to come, we had no doubts that He would take care of the details. However, if we allowed ourselves to think about it, it would be overwhelming. We had to live day by day, and often moment by moment, not thinking about what would or could happen. We knew we just had to do what needed to be done for the time being. We would have to do our part and let Him do His part.

About the second week in August, we headed back to our new home—our two-bedroom apartment in Memphis. We realized that we needed to get used to the idea that we *lived* here now, and that we were going to have to live as a split family. Saying goodbye was so difficult, and I was fearful it wouldn't get any easier. Plus, now there were no visitors to help me. I was on my own with Abby's care, and I was also feeling the effects of my last month of pregnancy.

We got back to the hospital and continued with blood tests and preparing for the next round of chemo. The next one would be high-dose methotrexate (HDM), and she would receive it two weeks in a row. It is called "high" dose because it is twelve times stronger than the amount given for patients with some other types of cancer. This would be her first dose of this chemo agent, so I didn't know what to expect. I prayed that she wouldn't be as sick as she was the first round. I knew it would be so very difficult to see her go through that again.

We had worked out the plan that Abby would go ahead and have the next three weeks of chemo as her protocol directed— first the two weeks of HDM, and then the cis/dox combo the third week. It would then be time for me to go home to have the baby as Abby recovered from that round of chemo. Skip's mom would come to stay with Abby at that time. Thankfully, she would have a break from her chemo regimen the following two weeks. We would then figure out a way to get Grandma and Abby home to be with the rest of the family after her counts came back up and she was cleared to leave. As it turned out, Skip's mom ended up staying to help with Abby for almost an entire month.

Meanwhile, my mom would travel down to Memphis to drive home with me so I wouldn't have to travel alone. She would also help with the other three kids while I was in the hospital, and then she would stay to help me after I got home. We were so thankful for both mothers being willing and able to help, especially since this seemed to be the only solution to our situation.

Well, the plan didn't go quite as we hoped. Abby's chemo was delayed because of high liver counts from the HDM. So now, she would be scheduled for her cis/dox combo, the one that made her so sick, *after* I needed to leave and when Skip's mom would be the only one there with her. I hated that for both Skip's mom and Abby because I remembered how tough it was on Abby the first time. I was worried about how Abby would handle being that sick without her mommy being there. She was excited about Grandma coming, so that helped me to feel better. My mother-in-law was willing to do whatever it would take to help out—she knew it wouldn't be easy, and she never made us feel that it would be too much for her.

The time was nearing that I would have to leave to go home. My mom and Skip's mom were headed to Memphis, and we would continue with our plan for me to go home to have the baby. Abby was so excited to think that she would have Mommy and both grandmas to herself! It was a lot of fun with the four of us being together.

As I prepared to leave, my heart was so heavy thinking about leaving Abby. I despised the thought that I wouldn't be there for her during her next round of chemo. I so desperately wanted to be there for Abby! I worried about the effects it would have on my mother-in-law to have to deal with her in such a terrible state. I just couldn't bear the thought of leaving my poor Abby!

When the time came for me to leave for home, Abby started crying, causing me to start crying. All I could do was hold her and tell her I would see her soon. Grandma would bring her down when she got better after her chemo, and she could see her new sister. I told her that I would not be leaving her if I didn't *have* to! It was so very hard on me to leave her like that, but I knew it wouldn't get easier. I had to go ahead and leave. Despite the tears and the overwhelming heartache of leaving my daughter, bewildered, I *had* to go.

I was thankful for the company of my mother on the trip home. If I would have had to travel that alone, I would have probably cried the whole way. As it was, I cried until we got well outside of Memphis. Even though I felt such pain in leaving her, I was also thankful for the care I knew she would receive while I was gone.

We got home with one day to prepare for the baby's arrival. I was excited to be home with Skip, Emma, Micah, and Zach, but part of my heart was still back in Memphis. It seemed so strange to be home without Abby—the house just didn't feel right. It just felt like there was something missing. I remember thinking that was odd because much of the time around our house, the kids are back in the bedrooms playing; but I could still feel her absence. I didn't like that feeling. I missed my Abby and felt she needed her mommy. I was overwhelmed because I couldn't be both places that I wanted to be.

On the other hand, I was about to have a baby! I was so excited about our new addition; it was just that the timing seemed inconvenient. I had wished there was an easier way to work it out, and that we could all be together at home like we should be.

Skip and I headed to the hospital early on the scheduled day for my induction. I was excited to be able to spend the day with just Skip, even under the circumstances. Abby was scheduled to go into the hospital the same day to get her chemo. Everything went pretty much as planned, and Zoe Ruth was born early that evening. She was a tiny six pounds, six ounces. I wasn't used to that, since all of my other ones had ranged from seven pounds, six ounces to seven pounds, thirteen ounces. She was beautiful. No Down syndrome, no club foot (though even now, she does turn her foot sideways, and I could see why they might have thought they saw a club foot), no kidney problems—just absolutely perfect! For the present moment, my world was complete as I held my little baby in my arms.

I found that having and recovering from a six pound-something baby was much easier than seven pound-something babies. Praise the Lord that He worked out the details. I would be well on my way to recovery when I headed back to Memphis in three weeks to care for Abby again, with my tiny newborn in tow.

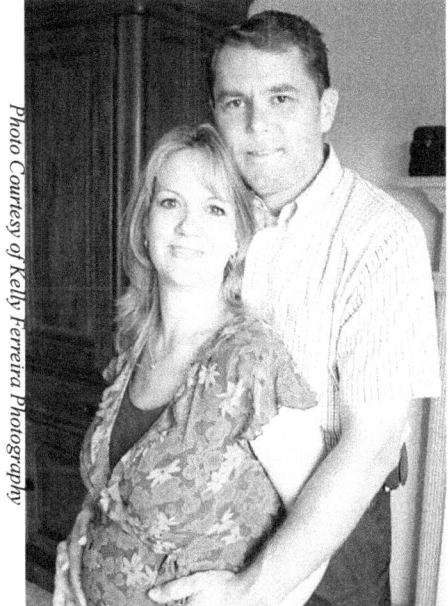

Talk about juggling rhinos—Abby's treatments, living miles apart, and a new baby?!

We called Skip's mom later on to see how Abby was doing. She was doing amazingly well considering her circumstances. She had significantly less nausea, and they were doing such a great job controlling her discomfort! She wasn't *nearly* as sick as she was the first time. Praise the Lord! *He* was taking care of her when I couldn't be there.

One thing that made me terribly sad, though, was that when I talked to Abby on the phone, she cried and said she missed me and wanted me. I realized it would be best for her to not talk to me; that way, she wouldn't miss me, making the situation easier on everyone. So, I didn't talk to her much after the first few days of being away. Because of this, she adjusted well to my being away. I still missed her tremendously though, and I couldn't wait for her to come home.

Grandma had done a good job of keeping Abby busy until she recovered enough to travel. After a slight delay, they were able to come home for that last week before having to go back to Memphis. The only way we could get them home was for Skip to drive up to get them and then drive straight back. It was a wonderful reunion, and Abby was so excited to see her new baby sister. We were once again able to enjoy being a full family—now a family of seven!

Emma, Micah, and Zach had been enjoying having Grandma and Mommy home. Emma was so excited about the new baby. She was a living doll to her. Micah was pretty excited about her too, but Zach really didn't pay too much attention to her either way. He was only three, so it didn't make too much sense to him; his life was upside-down anyway.

That was also the time we needed to address the vehicle issue. We didn't need to make a decision now because we already had a car that seated six and a car that seated five. We thought it would be nice, though, for the times that we were together to not have to drive separately, taking two vehicles wherever we went. We already coveted *any* time that we had together, even if it was just in the car.

I was supposed to leave to go back to Memphis with Abby on the third Monday in September; but because I was sick and needed to go on antibiotics, we got permission to cancel Abby's appointments and stay home until Wednesday. That Tuesday, Skip had an appointment at one of his listed properties considerably north of our home. On his way, he saw a van on the side of the road that said "for sale." We looked at it, and we decided it would be perfect for us. Now we could all ride together.

The Lord worked it out that we could get the vehicle we needed before I went back to Memphis. We were amazed to watch as He continued to provide and work out the details for us. He continued to be faithful and take care of us as we trusted in Him throughout this difficult journey.

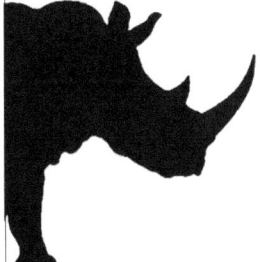

Family of Three?

Family of Three?

So, back to Memphis we went—continuing along our faith-building journey. Abby, Zoe, and I would need to get used to our new little family of three for the time being. We were the new "Tennessee Three." We got the apartment set up with the new baby things and prepared to continue Abby's appointments and treatments. Going to Memphis this time seemed more permanent. We didn't have any more scheduled breaks or distractions to look forward to, but thankfully we would find stability and blessings along the way.

Because Abby had been having a considerable amount of pain in the middle of her femur, they scheduled an appointment for an x-ray shortly after we got back to the hospital. They told us that they could then decide whether or not she could get her cast off. Well, the x-ray showed that the top of her cast was putting pressure just above the fracture, which wasn't healing, and that was causing the pain. Because her bone had deteriorated to the point that her leg could not be stable, they decided that she would need to keep her leg in a cast until her surgery. They would have to do something different with her cast to relieve the pressure and pain.

Instead of getting that despised cast off, they added to the top of it, extending it all the way to the top of her thigh. It was pretty bulky at the top, since they casted over top of the old one. Poor Abby; she was already tired of having to wear the cast and maneuver on her crutches. This news was not what she wanted to hear. The cast held her back so much from being able to play and act like a normal kid. She wanted to be able to enjoy the playground, but she couldn't with her cast and crutches. Throughout the previous weeks, she had learned to maneuver with her crutches very proficiently; and she was able to get around pretty quickly.

Abby was very noticeable as she moved through the halls of the hospital with her bright pink cast, her bright pink crutches, and her little bald head. Even at St. Jude, she stuck out and was very recognizable—it seemed that everyone knew who Abby was, or at least they knew about the little girl with the pink cast and pink crutches. At first, there had been this very pregnant mother with this new patient hobbling around on her crutches, which drew attention. Now that we were back, we had a newborn. This drew even more attention!

Trying to ease the hardship of our separation, Skip brought the kids up early in October for a long weekend. He took me to a church just across the border in Mississippi, where we had previously come into contact with the pastor. He had come to the hospital during Abby's visit for her first round of chemo. We were friends with his brother and sister-in-law, and they had told him about us. Because I hadn't been brave enough to go by myself to find it, I was thankful that Skip took me that Sunday. Throughout my stay in Memphis, I attended that church whenever I was able. They loved Abby and prayed consistently for her throughout her treatment. I know God provided them for us, as they were continually a blessing to us.

Thankfully, the Lord had blessed our real estate business over the summer with several good closings, especially after our slow start to the year. This was a big change from the two winters before, and we were so thankful for the Lord's provision, giving us the freedom to be together some during this separation in our family.

Abby went on with her chemo treatments, and we were expecting her surgery to be around the ten-week point in her protocol. This originally would have put it toward the end of September. Because of delays in her chemo and the doctors' schedules, we were informed that her surgery wouldn't be until the second week in December. This concerned us because of other problems that could come with a delayed surgery date.

The issues Abby was having with her leg concerned her doctor. He feared that the chemotherapy wasn't working because of her additional pain and swelling. At one point, he talked about having to put her on another chemo agent if these three weren't working, adding three months to our stay. Those were not words that I wanted to hear! Because he also did not want to wait that long for her surgery, he said he would do what he could to move it up.

Abby had been such a trooper about wearing the cast, but I knew that she was already so tired of having it on. Her MRIs showed more and more deterioration, and her femur was now actually completely fractured and terribly misaligned. We had been told that since her femur had completely broken, the cancer may spread, since it wasn't contained inside the bone any longer. That, along with the concern of muscle loss from her leg being in a cast for so long and her obvious discomfort, made us all ready to get her surgery out of the way. After some rearranging of schedules, they decided to schedule her surgery just before Thanksgiving. We decided to take the soonest possible date, so we went ahead with that plan.

Meanwhile, we lived day to day with our appointments and chemo treatments. We went to the hospital pretty much every weekday for appointments, and we were even in the hospital over some weekends. We had our ups and downs with Abby's blood counts, transfusions, and chemistries, as would be expected during chemo treatments. The Lord continued to see us through the day-to-day details.

Throughout this time, Abby had many great opportunities, including photo shoots for press and mailings, promotional materials for groups supporting St. Jude, the St. Jude calendar, and their product catalog. She also enjoyed getting to meet many people—some famous, as well as some regular, wonderful people there to support St. Jude. She also helped in videos used for fundraising commercials, thank-you's for supporters, as well as a television network that was premiering St. Jude in a fundraising telecast. I was thankful for the opportunities to help give back a little for what St. Jude had done for Abby and for our family!

At the beginning of November, we were able to go home to visit for a few days. We had been asked to share Abby's story at the St. Jude Celebrity Golf Tournament in Destin, Florida, while we were home. We gladly accepted the invitation and spent the weekend over in Destin.

Family of Three?

It was an exciting experience to attend the benefit and auction and to be able to thank people personally who supported St. Jude's efforts to help Abby and children like her. Because of some disorganization on our part and confusion with the schedule for the evening, Skip ended up on stage telling Abby's story, while I went to find her. About the time Skip was finishing up, I brought Abby up front. When she came up on stage, the whole room gave her a standing ovation! I was extremely touched at their graciousness to her. That was a moment of awe as we saw the amazing support for our little girl, and the tears welled in my eyes. Our trip to Destin was a nice weekend getaway, with many great memories, that we enjoyed together as a family before going back to St. Jude for her surgery. The Lord blessed us with some of these wonderful moments!

The week before her surgery was another one of those highlights. Abby was asked to give a tour of the hospital to television host Hoda Kotb which would be aired on NBC's Today Show the week of Thanksgiving. Abby thoroughly enjoyed that, and she was all smiles the entire time. She showed Hoda around on her little crutches, moving through the hospital hallways with ease. They invited her and the whole family to come to New York to spend a few days the following week. They wanted her to be on the show live, but we sadly had to turn the opportunity down because Abby's surgery was scheduled that week. There was no postponing that! It was disappointing, but we were thankful that her surgery was finally here. We were also grateful for the gracious invitation that we had been given.

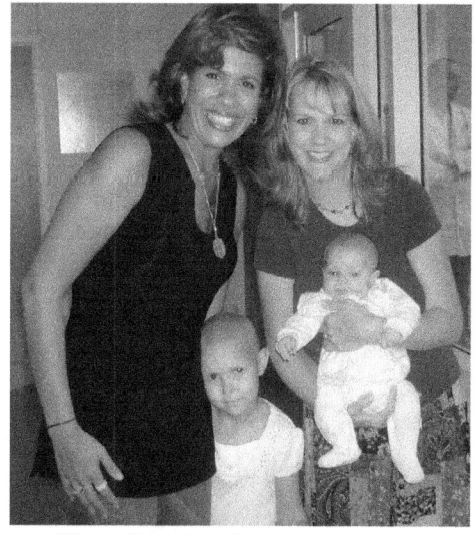

We really enjoyed our opportunity to meet Hoda.

God proved Himself to be our stability in our highly unstable world throughout these periods of unknowns and valleys. We were thankful each day for the little blessings we received in many different ways.

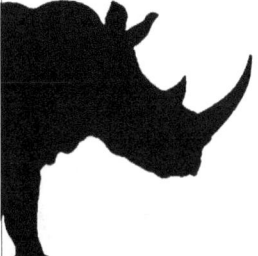

A Brave
Little Girl

A Brave Little Girl

The Lord continued to give us grace, guidance, and peace as we worked out the details for Skip to come up and spend a couple of weeks with me during Abby's surgery. Skip would then stay through his birthday so we could be together as a family for that as well. Skip's sister would keep Emma, Micah, and Zach in the Nashville area while Skip stayed in Memphis with me.

I was thankful for the support I had with Skip there throughout those two weeks. Skip, Emma, Micah, and Zach came to Memphis, and

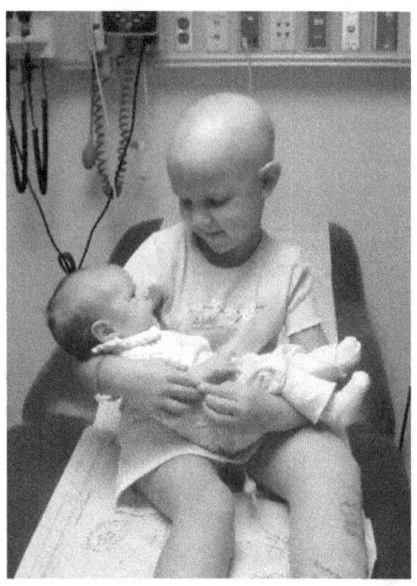

Our "normal" life at St. Jude

our brother-in-law made the trip over to pick up the kids and take them back to Nashville. There was nothing I would have liked better than to keep the family together, but we knew it was for the best that they were not there. We needed to focus on making it through the next few days.

It made sense for Emma, Micah, and Zach to stay with Skip's family during this time. Abby would be better off without the extra commotion that three kids would bring to a hospital room. Plus, we knew the kids would find it hard to understand what was going on with Abby. We wanted to protect them from that as well. We also needed to be able to stay together at the Target House, which would mean only four of us in Memphis. The environment would be much happier and lighter for the kids to be able to stay and play with their cousins. I was thankful that we had this option and that his sister was gracious in providing this help.

Abby handled everything in stride, and she didn't really show any anxiety as we prepared for her surgery. She had gotten so tired of that cast that she was ready to have her surgery just to get rid of it! A day or so before her surgery, Abby was in the hospital cafeteria explaining to Micah what would happen during her surgery. She told him that they would cut her leg open, cut out her bone, and put in a fake bone in its place. She said that it would hurt a little, but she would be okay. She then turned to me and quietly said that she really did think it would hurt *a lot*, but she didn't want to scare Micah. I thought it was so precious and sweet that she was thinking more of Micah than of herself, even though she was the one who would be going through the surgery. She kept an amazing outlook throughout the preparation for surgery and even afterward.

The night before her surgery was full of mixed emotions. It was so difficult to think about what Abby would have to go through the following day, and what she would have to endure during recovery. But she *had* to have the surgery. They *had* to get the cancer out of her body. I was ready for her to be able to move on; she was ready to move on. She'd had her cast on for four months. We were tired of her not being able to take a normal bath and being held back in so many ways by the awkward cast. We wanted her to be able to play again like a six-year-old should play. We knew it would still be quite some time before she would be able to, but at least this was a step in that direction. It was difficult to watch her have to give up the ability to play like she normally did before she was diagnosed with osteosarcoma. We also had to say goodbye to Emma, Micah, and Zach that night, again feeling the loss and separation associated with our family not being together. Abby was also very disappointed that she wasn't able to go over to stay with the cousins; she was feeling left out of the excitement. There was so much going on in our hearts and minds.

Our brother-in-law headed over from Nashville to pick up the kids, and we spent that evening with Scot and Jill as a family. Their love and concern was so evident and appreciated as we thought about the events taking place the next day. Before heading back to the Target House to prepare for the next day, we were able to enjoy a relaxing evening together. Shortly after the kids left for Nashville, it was time for us to head to the apartment—the events were moving ahead whether we liked it or not.

There was plenty of fear associated with the unknown. The doctor had previously told us that they wouldn't know if the chemo was working until her surgery. We were afraid to find out that it hadn't been working, thus adding three months to this already lengthy journey. He had also said that they wouldn't know until going in if they would be able to save her leg. If there wasn't enough good tissue to work with, she would have to have a full amputation. Would we find her after the surgery without a leg at all? How difficult would her life be as such a young child with only one leg? Fears and questions tended to swell as we contemplated what we may be facing the next day. However, we still felt a peace that God was in control. No matter the outcome, the grace that we would be given would be sufficient.

The plan for her surgery was to remove the tumor with enough of a margin to make sure that they removed the entire cancerous area. She also had a small skip lesion, a small tumor, above the main tumor in her leg. That would cause them to have to take more of her femur than they had originally thought. They would then insert an internal prosthesis called a Repiphysis®. The wonderful thing about this prosthesis was that it would grow with Abby. It would give her the opportunity to keep her leg without having to have future surgeries to lengthen it as she grew. This device has an internal spring and an electromagnetic field that serves as a locking mechanism used to adjust the length of the prosthetic "bone." We were so thankful that this was an option for Abby and that she could very possibly be able to keep her leg!

There was nothing we could do to help her through the surgery. In our hearts we wished so much that we could take it all away or that it could be one of us to go through it for her. It is a helpless feeling as a parent to know that there is nothing you can do to take away your child's pain.

Thankfully, we knew that the Lord cared more for Abby than we did ourselves. Nothing would happen to Abby that He didn't allow. There was such peace knowing that our God was by our side, and He was big enough to handle it for us.

November 20th came, and Abby was scheduled for surgery first thing in the morning. Our little Abby was in surgery for five hours, where they removed her knee and most of her femur. They kept us updated throughout the stages of surgery, but the moments and the events of that day are such a blur for me. I remember highlights, but I do not remember much of what happened throughout that day. I vaguely remember sitting in the waiting room, going to see her during recovery where the anesthesia had made her sick, and then how terrible she looked from the effects of the surgery.

After the surgery, our minds whirled with gratefulness as we stood by her bedside. They had resected (removed) the tumor, placed the internal prosthesis in place of the femur and knee, allowed Abby to recover from anesthesia, and brought Abby to her hospital room. We were able to be with her through recovery and as they took her to her room. Her pain was well-controlled with a nerve block as well as by intravenous medications. More than anything at this point, we were thankful that she still had her leg.

They also previously told us that she might need to spend a day or two in ICU initially, depending on how her surgery went; but they released her to a normal room. Her doctor said the surgery went "picture perfect" with no complications. God again provided the grace for us to make it through!

Poor little Abby looked so pitiful—all swollen and groggy from the anesthesia. She was barely recognizable. She had a large bandage covering her entire leg, which was extremely swollen. It was sad to see her in that condition. She had tubes and lines everywhere it seemed, but the Lord continued to take care of her. She had an amazingly problem-free surgery; and aside from needing a blood transfusion, which isn't unusual for a surgical patient, a problem-free recovery.

As they decreased the bandage on her leg over the next couple of days, it was cute to see how happy Abby was to actually be able to touch and feel the back of her leg. She thought it felt so good to be able to rub her leg after being in a cast for so long! I was thankful to be able to see her cute little foot again. I'll always love seeing that foot because it can constantly remind me how thankful I am that she has that foot, and it was spared the amputation that was a possibility.

Her doctor prepared us that at some point in the future, something *will* go wrong with her leg—it may be something big, or it may be something small, but it will go wrong. So far, she has remained stable without any complications. I know we have a very long time to go with Abby's leg in its current state, and

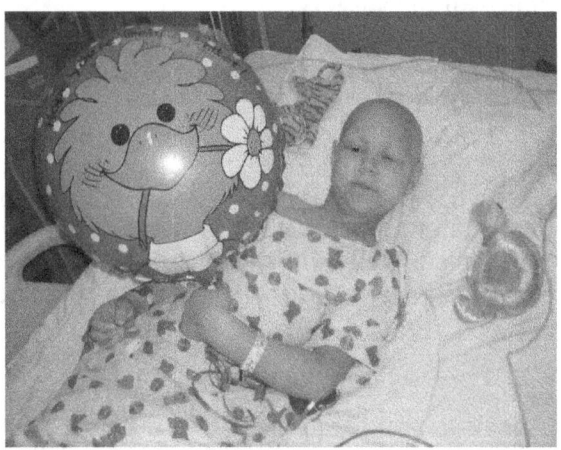
Abby just hours after her surgery.

problems could easily arise with the weaknesses of this early-generation prosthesis. I am thankful, however, to have made it this far with so much progress and no difficulties. I guess the doctor should have said that something will go wrong if the Lord allows it.

Abby also started her long journey of physical therapy following her surgery. She would need to learn to walk again. Her muscles were weak from not using them for the four months she was in a cast; and the muscles, tendons, nerves, and veins were disturbed from the surgery and needed to heal. She had a big hurdle to overcome to get back up on her feet and walk without her crutches again. She would have physical therapy three hours a week to regain range of motion and the ability to walk. This was a journey that lasted far past her time at St. Jude.

Abby spent about five days in the hospital following her surgery, and she was given about a week to recover before they started her chemo again. I am amazed at what her little body went through. She lost almost 10 pounds since we arrived in July, which was about 20 percent of her total body weight prior to her diagnosis. At times, I would find myself wondering how much her body could take. Overall, she just didn't look well with dark circles under her eyes and pale skin. She didn't look like herself, besides the obvious fact that she didn't have hair. She just looked sickly.

We looked forward to her recovering and getting back to normal. We were ready for her to be healthy and whole again, and we knew it would have to be the Lord who would get her to that point. He had proven Himself faithful to this point in providing the strength, grace, and peace that we needed; and we had no reason to believe that He wouldn't see us through the remainder of the journey.

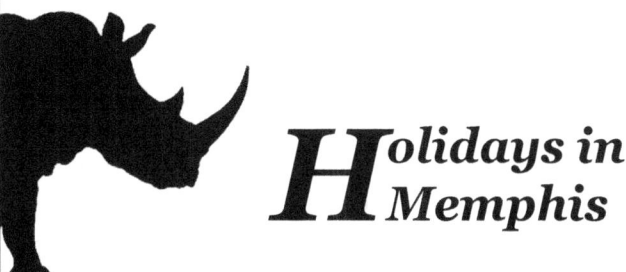

*H*olidays in Memphis

Holidays in Memphis

Throughout these months, the Lord was constantly reminding us of the value in our family relationships. We learned so much about not taking these special relationships for granted from day to day, as you never know what the future holds. The holiday season is always a special time for families, and we were looking forward to what this season would hold for us, even in our unusual circumstances.

Abby was released from the hospital a day or two before Thanksgiving, just five days after the surgery to remove the tumor in her leg. Since we had Thanksgiving Day free of appointments and the kids were only three hours away in Nashville, we decided it would be nice to be together for Thanksgiving as a family, since Abby's doctors cleared us to go. Unfortunately, the day before Thanksgiving, two of the cousins came down with strep throat. We weren't able to go to Nashville as planned. Since we couldn't risk exposing Abby to strep throat because her immune system was weakened, we spent Thanksgiving apart.

That was hard on us, but at least we knew we'd be able to see the kids soon. We had so much to be thankful for, yet it was disappointing to not be able to spend the holiday together as a family. We spent Thanksgiving with Scot and Jill's family, and we had a special day with some delicious food!

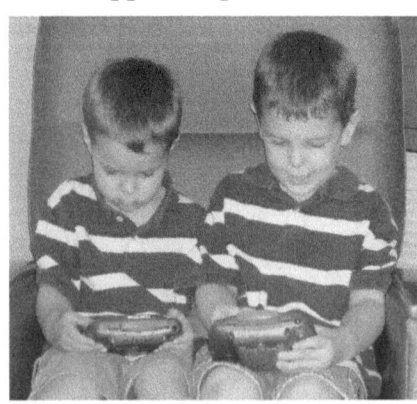
Keeping Zach (left) and Micah (right) busy at the hospital

Early in December, we were able to be back together to spend some time celebrating Skip's birthday. My sister-in-law had done a great job keeping Emma, Micah, and Zach healthy so they weren't sick when it came time to come back over to Memphis. We were so thankful that we didn't have to keep Abby away from them, since they didn't get strep throat. We were able to enjoy some days together as a family before the "Florida Four" had to go home. The separation was still difficult, but this time we knew it would only be for a couple of weeks.

The first week in December, we were asked to go to New York City for Abby to ring the opening NASDAQ bell on behalf of St. Jude Children's Research Hospital. The news of being able to go to New York City for such a special event came as an exciting surprise! Abby's doctors approved the trip, so Abby, Zoe and I planned to fly to New York for a couple of days—this would be a new experience for all three of us!

Abby, with her new prosthesis, was rather enthusiastic about being able to make the detectors in the airport "beep" when she went through. I wasn't quite as excited about it because of the extra security measures; but truthfully, I couldn't help but smile because Abby found humor in it. All in all, it worked out fine because Abby's situation was fairly obvious just by looking at her—with her little bald head and crutches. We were on our way to New York.

We flew into Newark, where they had a car waiting to take us to the hotel. As we arrived in the city, we were amazed at all of the tall buildings, the lights and sounds, and the extreme amount of traffic. It made me thankful I didn't have to drive in New York City! We arrived at our hotel excited about being able to spend these two days in a new place, unlike anywhere we had been before.

Because she just had chemo a few days before, Abby had some difficulty with nausea as well as pain in her leg while we were in New York. Because Abby wasn't feeling very well and I wasn't brave enough to take my two little girls out alone in New York City, we stayed in the hotel quite a bit.

We did, however, enjoy ourselves by visiting NASDAQ and participating, live, in ringing the opening bell. We also had the opportunity to visit the three-story Toys 'R Us store, as well as the shops and restaurant of the hotel. Overall, we had a great time and loved seeing the lights and hearing the sounds of New York City.

We were thankful for these fun and unique distractions as they came about—a little good that we were able to experience through the bad. We saw them as a blessing because we knew we would never have had many of these opportunities had our circumstances been different.

Skip, Emma, Micah, and Zach were able to come back up a few weeks later for Christmas break. Skip loaded the kids and drove to Memphis to spend Christmas with us. Over these months, many miles were traveled in our driving back and forth to visit each other.

We would have liked nothing more than to be able to spend Christmas—Zoe's first Christmas—as a family in our own home, with our *own* Christmas tree, around our *own* fireplace. Under the circumstances, that just wasn't an option for us this year. Abby was required to stay in Memphis for the six weeks following her surgery to watch for any complications, and she also needed to stay on schedule with her chemo.

The Lord blessed us that Christmas in spite of our location. We were all together. This was the best gift, considering our circumstances. Abby was with us, and her prognosis was good. We had learned a short time earlier that Abby's chemo *was* working; they told us that the tumor had shown nearly one-hundred percent necrosis! That meant that the tumor was almost completely killed by the chemo before her surgery. We would not have an extended stay after all. That just served as an extra blessing from the Lord throughout the holiday season.

A very dear friend of mine, along with her family, put together a couple of large boxes of gifts for the kids, Skip, and me. They were so thoughtful and gracious to us, and we were appreciative of their kindness and caring about our family's Christmas from so far away. The Lord used them to be such a blessing to us in spite of our Christmas away from home. They didn't have to do that, especially since they had families of their own to buy gifts for. We were so grateful for their generosity and kindness.

In fact, throughout the months that we lived in Memphis, many people sent cards and packages to Abby. As Abby opened each one, there was such delight and happiness for both of us

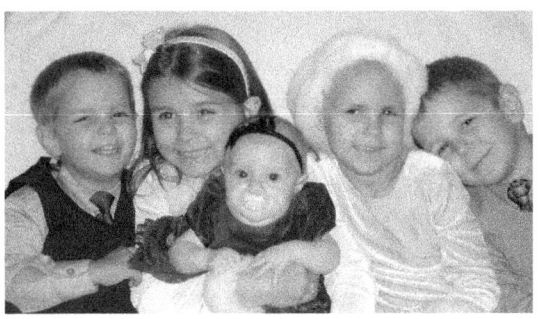

Christmas at the Target House

that people were thinking of her. It was special for me, as her mother, to be able to enjoy the smiles that they brought—as there were times that Abby's smiles weren't so easy to come by.

The Target House was also gracious to each of the resident families during Christmas, since they were all away from home for the holidays. They provided gifts for each of the children. Staying at the Target House throughout our time in Memphis was a comfortable home away from home. We were treated extremely well the entire stay. It was also amazing to be able to meet the other families living there that were going through similar circumstances.

When the time came for the kids to go back to school, Abby had a few days open in her protocol so we could go home with Skip and the kids. We got to spend the first few days in January at home. We were so thankful for the opportunity since this was our first time home in over two months.

Overall, we had a very good Tennessee Christmas. The Lord blessed us beyond measure during these days together. Our greatest gift, aside from the gift of Jesus Christ as we celebrated His birth, was the gift of being together!

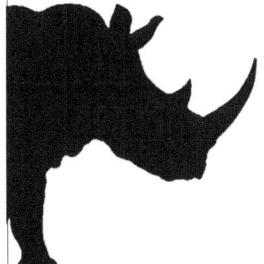

The Sun Shines Brighter

The Sun Shines Brighter

We headed back to Memphis with the major milestones behind us, and the end was coming into sight. Our current focus was to continue with our daily appointments, so we could reach the end of this journey and our lengthy family separation. We still had about three months of chemotherapy left.

Because Micah's birthday was coming up toward the middle of February and my birthday was a few days after that, we decided to try to make plans to be together during that time. Since they had already missed so many days, we realized that it wouldn't be possible for Skip to take the kids out of school again. As long as there weren't any delays in her chemo, it looked like Abby would have a twelve-day break in her schedule around that time, so we planned to go home to be with Micah for his birthday and stay for mine as well.

Families in long-term housing are typically only allowed to be away seven days at a time. In order to be gone that long, we had to request special permission from the housing department, as well as from the doctors. When they approved our request, we were elated. Abby was able to stay on schedule for her chemo for the most part, and we were excited that the plan was working. We would be able to go home!

The Friday we had planned to go home, we went in for Abby's scheduled lab draw to check her blood counts—the last thing we needed to do before leaving town. Abby had been telling everyone all day that we were going home. Because she had her chemo a couple of days before, and her counts would be on their way down, they needed to be monitored regularly. After receiving the results, they told us that Abby's ANC (absolute neutrophil count—in other words, her body's ability to fight sickness or infection) was only 100. For anything under 500, they advise patients to stay close to the hospital in case they get sick or run a fever because immediate treatment would be necessary. They said we should stay in Memphis, since traveling would be strongly discouraged.

As badly as I wanted to go home anyway despite the advice to stay, Skip and I decided that Abby, Zoe, and I should just stay put because it wasn't worth the risk to travel with Abby's low counts. Unfortunately, Zach had an upper respiratory infection, meaning Skip and the kids would not be able to come up to visit us. We were heartbroken! We were packed and ready to go. Abby had even gotten Micah a few things for his birthday. Our excitement instantly turned to overwhelming disappointment. Tears were abundant on both Abby's and my part.

Her doctor told us we could come in for a lab draw on Sunday because he knew we were planning to go home. We all knew this was a long shot because Abby's counts were still dropping and would probably be even *lower* by then—her bone marrow was so tired from the months of chemo. We were sure that they would be zero by Sunday. We would not be able to be home for Micah's birthday, which was Monday. It had only been a couple of days since her chemo, and her ANC had already dropped to 100. It was hopeless to think we'd be able to go at all, between Zach being sick and the length of time it would take for her counts to rebound.

Well, Sunday morning came, and we went to the hospital to have her labs drawn. Abby didn't even want to hear what the results were, so she plugged her ears to avoid the disappointment, just waiting to see my expression. To our amazement, her ANC was 700! They had previously cleared her to travel at anything over 500. I can only explain it as a *miracle* that it had rebounded to 700! At this point, Abby had been on chemotherapy for several months; and as expected, her body had been taking longer and longer to recover. This sudden jump in her ANC came as an absolutely amazing surprise. Abby and I could not get over our excitement! We got to go home after all! We went straight back to the apartment to pack and start for home.

Because Micah was disappointed that we were not able to come home for his birthday, as were Skip and the other two kids, Abby and I decided that it would be fun to surprise them. We were giddy with excitement the whole way home as we anticipated the surprise of our arrival. We really wondered if we could pull it off, but it worked out perfectly. None of them even suspected that we were on our way home. Being able to go home was so much fun, especially after fearing that we most likely wouldn't be able to go. We got home Sunday evening, just in time to be together for Micah's birthday the next day. The surprise on Skip, Emma, Micah, and Zach's faces was unforgettable!

Besides the fact that her counts were dropping and should not have been rebounding, one of the reasons that I believe it was a miracle for us to be able to go home (and that it *had* to be the Lord who caused her ANC to be 700 that day) was that her ANC had dropped back down to 400 when we had her labs drawn the following Tuesday—just two days later. It was truly amazing how the Lord obviously provided the way for us to go home. We spent the next nine days at home together as a family. Micah's birthday, as well as mine, was wonderful because we were together as a family.

Abby had about six weeks of chemo left. As the time was drawing nearer to go home for good, it was getting more difficult to leave Skip. I was tired of being apart and just wanted to get everything back to normal. We wanted to spend time together, but the phone was our only option. It was so hard to have enough to say. I longed to be able to spend time with him without having to say anything. A long-distance relationship just wasn't what we had in mind.

I also felt that I was drawing further away from Emma, Micah, and Zach. It had been so long since I had been able to be their Mommy. I missed them so much! I couldn't wait to get back to the point that I was a part of their everyday lives. Nine months is a very long time to miss from a child's life. And while I was missing out on those three, Skip was also missing out on Abby and Zoe. He missed so much of getting to know Zoe, as she was developing so quickly at that stage.

We found that discipline was also very difficult to balance during our separation. It wasn't easy to know where to draw the line while we were single parents. It was hard to be the sole disciplinarian while our children were going through such a time of instability in their lives. It also wasn't easy to be a disciplinarian with the kids that we didn't get to see very often. We longed for the time together to be nothing but pleasant. We just had to trust that the Lord would direct and that everything would get back to normal after our separation was finally over.

We were also concerned about getting back together as a family after this long separation and how it would affect us. I had developed my own independence by only having to think of myself and the two children I had, and Skip had developed his own independence in taking care of the home and the other three kids. He had his way of doing things at home that I wasn't used to, and I wondered if it would be a stressor when the time came for us to live together again.

There had also been so much strife between Emma and Abby during our visits together. Abby just wanted the friendship of her big sister while they were together; but Emma had been jealous of Abby and the good things she was able to get and experience during this time. This caused a lot of arguing and bitterness between them. I was worried about how that would work out once we came home. I prayed that they would end up getting along when the time came.

Over the past months of treatments, Abby's body was wearing down. I longed for the end and for the time that her poor, dilapidated body could regain its normal function and health. She had lost so much weight because she wasn't able to eat much due to her taste changes, nausea and vomiting, and the horrible mouth sores. She had needed several transfusions to boost her blood counts, and she had frequent bloody noses—some of which were severe. I was ready for my little girl to be back in a normal state of health and regain the carefree life that a child should have. We were almost there!

In March, Abby was presented with another opportunity to give back to St. Jude when they invited her to shoot a commercial with Sara Evans for the St. Jude Dream Home Giveaway. We made the trip to Nashville where Abby enjoyed participating in a photo shoot with Sara, and then the two of them went through the process of shooting the television commercial. It turned out great, and many people told me that they had seen Abby's picture as they entered Lowe's or many other stores promoting the St. Jude Dream Home Giveaway. It has been neat to hear of all of the different times that friends saw Abby either on these posters, in commercials, in the Math-a-Thon book, in the calendar, or in the catalogs for the St. Jude Gift Shop. I am thankful that Abby had the ability to help out in these ways to promote St. Jude and to give back at least a little for all of the wonderful care she received as a patient.

Finally, the time came that Abby was finished with her chemo! March 27, 2009 was Abby's final chemotherapy treatment. Oh, what a feeling that was! She had her "no mo' chemo" party while she was in the hospital. She was given a t-shirt and balloons, and all of her nurses came in to sing to her and throw confetti. It was a big deal, and she was all smiles!

The first week in April, Abby got to represent St. Jude patients when AOL came to the hospital to present computers to the hospital for use by the families. They asked me to tell Abby's story to the AOL representatives as they toured the hospital, and I was more than willing to share the wonderful things St. Jude had done for Abby. Abby then participated in a formal presentation in the hospital as the idea and the computers were presented. She enjoyed being in the spotlight.

Soon thereafter, Abby finished with her final evaluations, and we got to go *home*! April 16th, nine months to the day from the start of Abby's battle with osteosarcoma, we were finally finished with this incredible journey. No more long-term separation! We were on our way home to be back together as a family.

A couple of days after we returned home, we had a "welcome home" party for Abby that was graciously hosted by the Drowsy Poet Coffee Company in our hometown. They had been very supportive of our family throughout these nine months, so we were excited about having the party there. It was wonderful to see many people after being away, and we were able to thank everyone in person for their love and prayers for our family. Many came out to show their love for Abby, and we were elated to spend such a special time together. Talk about cloud nine!

Here we were with our lengthy journey behind us, surrounded by wonderful people who cared about us.

The Lord was so good to Abby throughout her battle with osteosarcoma. She maintained such a great attitude throughout her journey, and now we seldom find her down. She was great about just going with the flow and doing whatever she had to, because she realized that there was no other option. She also trusted the fact that we wouldn't have allowed all of this to happen to her if we had any other choice. She knows the Lord has been so good to her. She has been a blessing, and it was amazing watching her throughout her journey. We have been blessed by God adding Abby to our family!

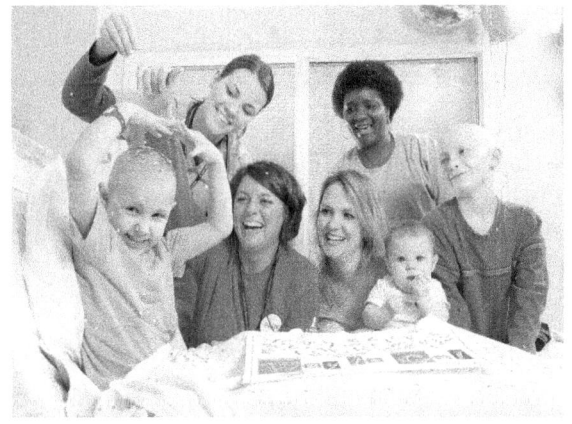

Abby's "No Mo' Chemo" Party at St. Jude

The blessings we received throughout those nine months were an incredible testimony of God's goodness even through the storms. The reuniting of our family was essentially seamless. My fears of the stress of getting back together were unfounded, as my wonderful husband was so patient with me. After a short time, it almost seemed like we hadn't even been apart, and it was great knowing that our journey was now just a memory.

The relationship between Emma and Abby was mended; and they are once again good friends, now that Abby is just one of the kids again. The bitterness and jealousy is gone. That was also an unfounded worry that I had. It is so silly when we worry about what might happen. The Lord is in control, and He will prove Himself faithful if we rely on Him. Their sisterly relationship is restored, and they enjoy having each other to play with. Emma has grown up so much and has matured quite a bit—she is my big helper at home. She is a joy to have around and has such a servant's heart. She loves people and it shows!

Micah and Zach have rebounded as well and have embraced getting back to normal. We have a wonderful relationship, and I am so thankful to be able to be a part of their lives every day again. They bring such joy and balance to our family. There is never a dull moment when the boys are around. They are growing so fast, and I know both will be tall, handsome young men before I know it. Micah is taller than Abby and outweighs her by ten pounds. Zach isn't far behind. The Lord blessed our family so much by adding our boys to it!

My questions of why the Lord gave Zoe to us during this time have been answered. She was such a blessing to us throughout that first year, and there hasn't been a day that she has not brought joy. He knew the timing would be just right, as she was a distraction to me. She helped draw some attention away from Abby, causing us to not completely spoil Abby. Even the sleepless nights were a blessing in disguise because they helped the time to go by so much more quickly.

Skip has remained steadfast through our whole journey. He loves the Lord, and it shows! I feel like I could go on

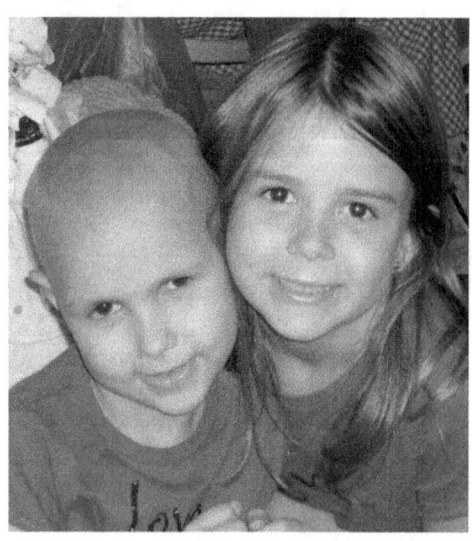

Sisters, happy to be reunited!

and on about him and not say enough. He is such a wonderful husband to me, and he is an amazing leader because he leads by example. He has the type of leadership that makes you *want* to follow him. It is not hard for me to want to be a submissive wife. I cannot imagine going through this journey with anyone else. God's hand was definitely there in placing Skip in my life to be my husband, soul mate, and best friend.

As a couple, Skip and I were brought closer through the trials. Sadly, this is not always the case as families go through similar circumstances. As I have thought about our relationship and how we've been able to stay so close, I can visualize us as pillars leaning toward each other. As the pillars lean toward each other, they come together at the top, but the weight of the trial cannot force them down. They have the support of each other. If the two pillars were leaning any other way but together, the weight would force them down, since they don't have the support of the other pillar. I'm thankful for our relationship, and I hope others can be encouraged by seeing that it is possible for a relationship to thrive through a storm.

I am blessed beyond measure with an amazing husband and family! Abby was now a two-time cancer survivor at age six, and we had many more lessons under our belt. We were extremely thankful to be at the end of this journey, but the lessons would prove to be invaluable as we continued on as a family.

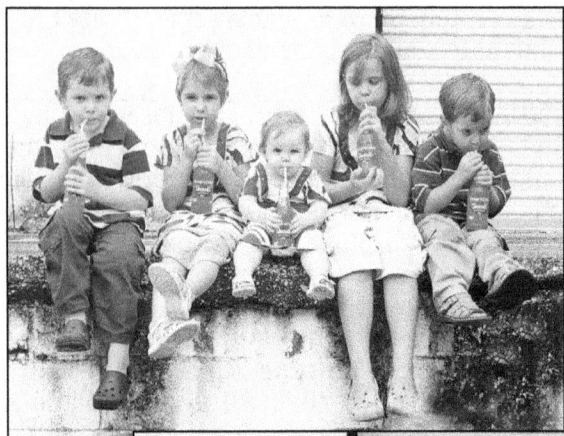

Photos Courtesy of Kelly Ferreira Photography

We were thankful to have our family back together again!

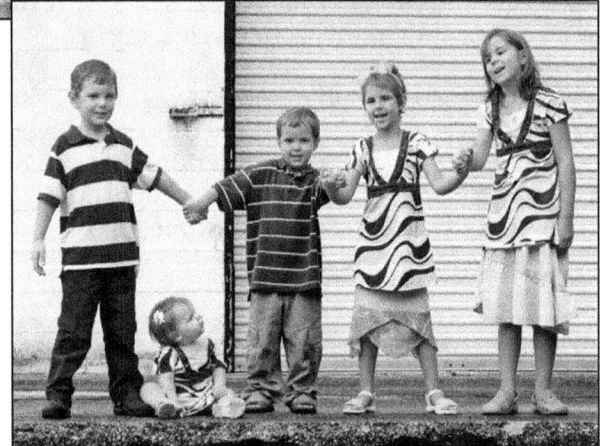

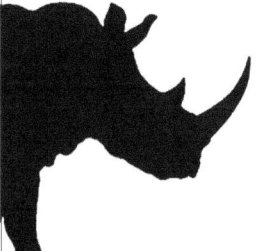

Lessons From Our Family

Lessons From Our Family

That is pretty much our lives through the end of Abby's treatments. Are we through with the trials? Most likely not, but we can continue to lean on the Lord and learn from the lessons that He gives us. We can continue to live as a testimony of His grace and be a light to those around us who do not know Him, as well as to those who need encouragement!

Through the difficult circumstances, the Lord has drawn me so much closer to Himself—causing me to actually be *thankful* for the storms! It's strange but true. It is amazing to see Him work in my life, as well as in the lives of my family. If we weren't tested by these storms, He would not be as evident to us.

Storms of life are similar to the idea of exercising. While no one—okay, mostly no one—really *enjoys* exercise, it is beneficial. It causes pain and discomfort, yet it still creates a positive outcome. Our natural tendency is to avoid the resulting pain and frustration. It is actually physically easier just to relax, but the lack of exercising our muscles makes our bodies weaker and more susceptible. The feeling after working out is exhilarating even though our bodies are crying out, "Please! No more!" The same is true of a storm.

Do I hope for more storms? No, but I do have comfort knowing that the Lord has helped us through our past difficulties. There is no reason for us to think that He will not continue to sustain us, no matter what arises in the future. Again, we can look to the light that we've seen in our lives to guide us through the dark paths.

Nothing is more comforting in our lives than knowing that the God of the universe, that sure Rock that cannot move even during the storms, has us in the palm of His hand. It is easier not to fear tomorrow because we can look back at the evidence in our lives that the Lord has held us up through the toughest times. Our greatest chance of survival through a storm comes through holding the hand of God! I don't know about you, but I feel a strong security with a God who has weathered and allowed every storm that has ever happened. Nothing happens without God's knowledge. He alone knows how to survive and even *thrive* in spite of these storms. I'm so thankful for these truths and how they have gotten me through the storms in my life, and I am thankful for a God who has never forsaken me. I have a confidence in my Lord that I couldn't possibly have in any person on earth!

God is the one, true Jehovah. He loves us beyond our imaginations, and He cares for us, even when it isn't apparent. God knows how to take care of our every need much better than we do. He even cares about the smallest details of our lives—even the details we think of as insignificant. Matthew 10:30 says that even the hairs on our head are numbered. Why does He care so much? Because He created us. As a parent loves his child, God loves us in that same way; but obviously, more perfectly. My life is a testimony of these attributes of my loving Heavenly Father.

The Lord has entrusted Skip and me with these storms to see if we would be found faithful throughout them. That is our truest hearts' desire—to remain faithful no matter what the storm and point the glory back to the Lord. We have realized that, in and of ourselves, we are nothing special; we are human. We can only be a testimony of God's grace to those that God places in our lives. He has never let us down. We do serve an amazing God!

If we look to the Lord, the storm doesn't look quite as bleak. By the grace of God, and only by His grace, we can weather *any* storm. We must keep our focus upward (toward God), instead of outward (into the storm). When we can find a way to share with others what we learned in our storm, and bring glory to the Lord, we can live a fulfilling life regardless of our circumstances.

We have learned it is necessary to prioritize the things that are important in our lives. God must be first and foremost. If He is not, we allow Satan to cause us to be ineffective in our Christian lives. Satan can use difficulties in our lives to lower us into despair and question our faith. This is right where Satan wants us—where the Lord cannot effectively use us.

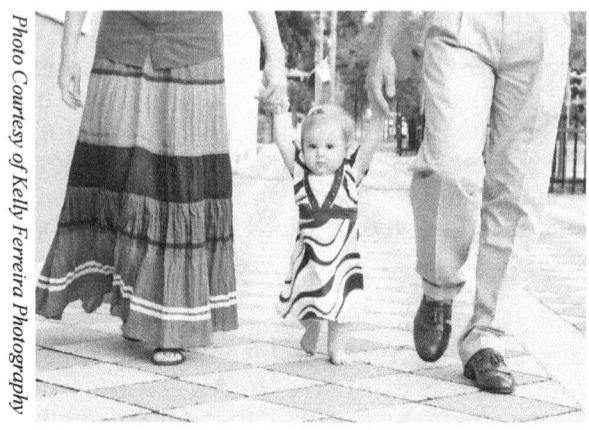

Our surprise blessing!

Our faith shouldn't only evidence itself through trials. The Lord should be the focus in our lives, even through our daily routines. We *need* Him every day, not just when we are going through hard times. Being a Christian isn't about hoping to have assurance of salvation while living a life void of anything spiritual. Being a Christian is *living* the Word of God and surrendering ourselves to it.

I learned many years ago that *God's way is the path of least consequences.* If God's Word says something specific about how we should live our lives, I can be sure that by listening to and obeying what it says, it will surely lead me down a much smoother path. For instance, Proverbs 22:7 says, "the borrower is servant to the lender." If we had heeded the wisdom presented in this verse, not wishing to be a "servant" in our finances, we would have made better choices when borrowing money. We could have avoided much of the heartache. The Bible can be used as a manual for life—it holds answers for pretty much any of life's situations. It teaches us how to live a life in peace with others and in a way that is pleasing to the Lord, bringing eternal benefits.

As storms approach, will we be found in a right relationship with the Lord, or will we have to get our hearts right before we can see His hand of blessing? Life is too short to live for anything but Christ. Our service to the Lord is the only thing that will last for eternity. Whether we are going through a storm or not, our relationship with our God and Creator should matter to us.

Where we keep our focus determines what we get out of life. Sadly, many times we don't choose to focus on the Lord. We may have to look inward to see what is standing in our way of a closer walk with Him. Bitterness, selfishness, anger, laziness, pride, or another personal sin may be the cause. For some, maybe the struggle is with more blatant and obvious sins. Some may think that a relationship with the Lord is too costly, but keeping these sins in our lives can only lead to lost blessings.

Our faith needs to be first and foremost in our lives. I have come across people who, after going through a trial in their life, question their faith. It doesn't have to be that way! You can look to God's Word for comfort in the promises that it gives. God's Word says in Hebrews 11:6, "But without faith it is impossible to please him." Faith in a loving God can get you through.

No matter how many things you place in your life to try to make you happy, you will never truly be satisfied until you have a relationship with the Lord. We are created with a "God-shaped" vacuum in our hearts. Until that void is filled with the Holy Spirit, we will continue searching for that fulfillment. My desire is to help you see the value in a relationship with the Lord. I want you to realize that in light of eternity, nothing is more important in our brief earthly lives than having a right relationship with the Lord and allowing Him to work in our lives. God's goodness then becomes so evident through the storms in our lives because we can feel His presence and His grace.

I learned something unique about God's grace through our journey of Abby's battle with osteosarcoma. A short time after we had come home, I was reading the journal that I had written during Abby's treatments. It was the strangest thing, but it seemed that I was reading someone else's story. I had to chuckle when I found myself feeling sorry for this person that I was reading about. The truth is, my strength throughout that time was coming from the grace God had provided for us each and every day of that storm. As I sat and read about our ordeal with Abby, it was a surreal experience because that same grace was no longer with me—I didn't need it anymore. I realized how much power was in the grace that was given to me in our time of need.

I have heard that grace can be likened to the manna in the Old Testament. God gave His people enough food in the form of manna each day. The people were free to gather as much as they needed, but only what they could use for the day. The next day there was new manna available, and the manna from the previous day was no longer food-worthy. Just like the manna, God gives us a fresh supply of grace to face each day.

As I continue along the journey that God has placed me on, I know that more storms will likely arise in my life; but I am thankful to know that I will always have God by my side to see me through them. That is my desire for you—to have the ability to experience His presence and grace throughout the storms in your life, no matter how many rhinos you are juggling.

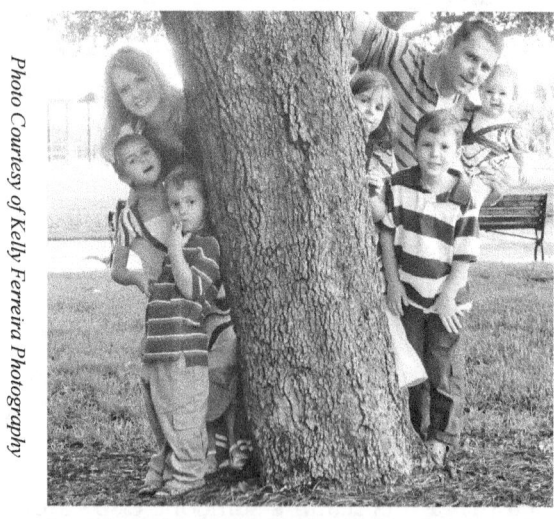

I am thankful for the family God has given me!

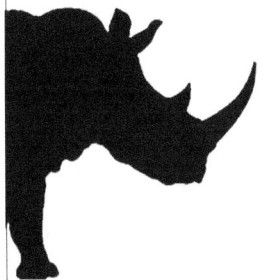

Sources of Inspiration

Sources of Inspiration

Some reading this may be in the middle of a storm. Actually, it is likely that many are currently facing a storm. The waves are crashing all around you, and you feel like there is no hope. I fear that when people are faced with these storms, they are left floundering and seeking answers to their fears and concerns. Based on my experiences, I am very certain that God is the answer to life's problems. I have experienced His grace first hand and know that it is readily available.

This section is meant to be a practical help for you to be able to reference the power and promises of God's Word as you face storms in your life. Sometimes we do not know where to turn or where to begin searching for answers. While this is not an all-inclusive guide to the many promises that God's Word offers, this will hopefully serve as a starting point and also as a quick reference for future storms that you will face. We need to be in the Word of God in order to know His promises for us. God's Word is of utmost importance in our sustenance and encouragement through the storms.

Many will question why the Lord allows us to go through a storm. We may not ever fully understand the reason why, but I do know that storms can be beneficial in our lives. They make us stronger and closer to God. I know that it is not God's plan for us to suffer, but He allows suffering and uses it in our lives. His original plan was to create man in His image for close fellowship and a relationship that is perfect. His creation was flawless—including no pain, problems, or storms—in a beautiful garden called Eden.

What does the Lord ask us to do through a storm? Simply pray, rest in Him, and give Him the glory. Because He knows that we can do nothing in our own power to help ourselves, He shows us that He is always there to go through the valley with us. How very comforting to know that He cares enough for us to carry us through! All we need to do is rely on Him.

Hebrews 4:16 says, "Let us, therefore, come boldly unto the throne of grace, that we may obtain mercy, and find grace to help in time of need." Isn't it amazing that God has a "throne of grace" that we can come to? This throne—this majestic, commanding seat—is available to us! It is the source of mercy— God's compassion on us as we deal with struggles in our lives. God knows we will have times of need, and I am so thankful for this throne that I can come to for the help of God Almighty! This verse also gives us the promise that we can come to the Lord in our time of need, knowing that He is the author of mercy. He also instructs us to come *boldly* to Him. We can come to Him expecting grace, if we can humble ourselves and ask for it. How do we get to this throne of grace? We find it on our knees, humbly asking God for His mercy—not because we deserve it, but because He is gracious. We can pray with the promise that He *will* help in our time of need.

I Corinthians 10:12-13 says, "Wherefore, let him that thinketh he standeth take heed lest he fall. There hath no temptation taken you but such as is common to man; but God is faithful, who will not suffer you to be tempted above that ye are able, but will, with the temptation, also make a way to escape, that ye may be able to bear it." This passage teaches us to realize that we cannot stand in the face of trials. If we have the confidence in ourselves to make it through, we had better be careful, because we will fall! No one has the power or the answers within themselves to handle life's tough situations. All we have to do is rest in Him, give the situation to Him, and leave it there. We can also know that God will limit the amount of trials that we face to only what we can handle. We are given the promise here that He is faithful to not give us too much!

He also gives us the comfort that we aren't the first to go through the fire, nor will we be the last. Others have walked in our shoes and have persevered in spite of storms, and by God's grace, we can too! Others will come after us on the same path, and with the Lord's help, they will make it through as well. Solomon said in Ecclesiastes 1:9, "There is no new thing under the sun." One hopeful outcome is that we will use our experience to reach out to help and encourage those who will go through the storm after we have.

The Lord promises that we can make it through. He will provide the way of escape that will free us from the clenches of the trial. We do, however, need to remember where the credit is due and give Him all the glory! I know I couldn't have made it through without the grace of God.

II Corinthians 12:9-10 says, "My grace is sufficient for thee; for my strength is made perfect in weakness. Most gladly, therefore, will I rather glory in my infirmities, that the power of Christ may rest upon me. Therefore, I take pleasure in infirmities, in reproaches, in necessities, in persecutions, in distresses for Christ's sake; for when I am weak, then am I strong."

These verses give encouragement in how to handle the storms in our lives. God's grace is sufficient—He will show His strength when we realize our weakness. When we sit back, look at the situation, and realize that we can do absolutely nothing to fix the problem, it is easy to realize that it will have to be the hand of God that brings us through to the other side. We can give God the glory because we can then see His power on our lives. That's a pretty amazing thing! We can be strong only in the strength of the Lord! He is the only way for us to have the strength to make it through.

This also explains why we can be thankful for the storms. As you experience trials, you are fully able to experience the power of Christ resting upon you. I believe it would be difficult to understand the full effect of Christ's power without going through times of distress. God uses suffering in our lives to make His power evident to us, allowing us to "glory in our infirmities."

Psalm 18:28-32, 46 says, "For thou wilt light my candle: the Lord my God will lighten my darkness. For by thee I have run through a troop; and by my God have I leaped over a wall. As for God, his way is perfect: the word of the Lord is tried: he is a buckler to all those that trust in him. For who is God save the Lord? or who is a rock save our God? It is God that girdeth me with strength, and maketh my way perfect. The Lord liveth; and blessed be my rock; and let the God of my salvation be exalted."

When we come to adversity or storms in our life, we need to realize that we cannot get it right on our own. We must turn to the Lord. God's way is perfect, and He promises His help if we trust in Him. He has always been faithful to help those in need, and we can be certain that He will continue to be faithful to us. After we find ourselves out of the valley, we need to be sure to give Him all of the glory.

I had stated earlier in this book: "I hadn't learned to fully rely on God for anything; I didn't have to rely on Him in my life free of storms." This truth allows me to see why God allows trials in our lives. Without trials and storms in our lives, we wouldn't need to learn to rely on Him and look to Him for guidance and provision. Thankfully, the Lord loved me enough to place tempests in my life. He cared enough to want to draw me closer to Himself through my storms. He taught me so much about myself and about who He is that I couldn't have learned otherwise. Putting purpose in the storms allows us to understand them and God's love so much better. He has a purpose for pain and suffering!

For me, it gives a new meaning to the verse in Romans 8:28 which says, "And we know that all things work together for good to them that love God, to them who are the called according to his purpose." Our first thought would be: "How can God use having a child with cancer for good?" Yet, the Bible states that *all* things work together for good. The good that comes from a situation like ours is that the power of God is manifested to us and through us. What an amazing situation we have found ourselves in!

We can use many other passages throughout the Bible for comfort and security throughout the storms. Through the leading of the Holy Spirit, we can turn to the Word of God for help throughout any of life's storms. It is important to know the promises given to us throughout the Word of God so we can claim them when needed.

The Book of Psalms is full of wonderful, amazing promises. There are also many promises in the New Testament as Jesus is teaching the world about Himself and His goodness. The emphasis in the following passages is mine.

Psalm 55:16-17 promises, "As for me, I will call upon God, and *the Lord shall save me*. Evening, and morning, and at noon, will I pray, and cry aloud, and *he shall hear my voice*."

Psalm 55:22 allow us to claim, "Cast thy burden upon the Lord, and *he shall sustain thee; he shall never suffer the righteous to be moved*."

Psalm 56:3-4 says, "What time I am afraid, I will trust in thee. In God I will praise his word, in God I have put my trust; *I will not fear* what flesh can do unto me." Then in verse 11, "In God have I put my trust; *I will not be afraid* what man can do unto me."

Psalm 57:2 states, "I will cry unto God most high; unto *God that performeth all things for me*."

Mark 10:27 says, "With men it is impossible, but not with God; for *with God all things are possible*."

Philippians 4:6-7 tells us, "*Be careful [anxious] for nothing;* but in every thing by prayer and supplication with thanksgiving let your requests be made known unto God. And the *peace of God, which passeth all understanding, shall keep your hearts and minds* through Christ Jesus." Then it continues on in verses 13 and 19, "*I can do all things through Christ* which strengtheneth me. But my *God shall supply all your need* according to his riches in glory by Christ Jesus."

The book of Isaiah also offers us hope in Isaiah 26:3-4, "Thou wilt *keep him in perfect peace*, whose mind is stayed on thee, because he trusteth in thee. Trust ye in the Lord forever; for in the *Lord Jehovah is everlasting strength*." Keep in mind the promise offered in verse 3 says that He will keep us in perfect peace, but we have to do our part in keeping our mind stayed on Him and trusting in Him. He will be our help and strength only if we allow Him to.

These are only a few of the passages that offer us promises as we trust in the Lord and as we go through difficult times. There are many more throughout God's Word that we could look to for help in times of trouble in our lives. As I contemplated passages to put in this book, I was overwhelmed by the many wonderful promises, and I realized that I couldn't possibly include them all. I encourage you to seek out more promises to arm yourself for storms that will come up or have come up in your life. Some will speak to you on a more personal level than they would to me. God's Word is amazing in that way!

The Lord *will* bless if we are faithful throughout the storms of life. We simply need to give it all to Him and rest in the fact that He is in control. He doesn't make any mistakes. He can and will see us through! Philippians 1:6 says, "Being confident of this very thing, that he which hath begun a good work in you will perform it until the day of Jesus Christ." And Ecclesiastes 3:11, 14 says, "He hath made every thing beautiful in his time...I know that, whatsoever God doeth, it shall be forever; nothing can be put to it, nor any thing taken from it; and God doeth it, that men should fear before him."

If you are in the middle of a storm, I pray that this testimony of how the Lord has worked in our lives will be an encouragement to you. He will work in anyone's life who is willing to allow Him to. Jesus Christ is the perfect Companion for us as we go through the trials in our lives. He, of all the people who have lived on this earth, knows so much about pain and suffering. He was described in Isaiah 53:3a, "He is despised and rejected of men, a man of sorrows, and acquainted with grief." Among many other storms, Jesus experienced the death of a very close friend, watched as some of His disciples openly betrayed Him, and kept silent as He, being innocent of any crime, was unjustly tortured, beaten, and hung to die on a cross. Therefore, He can relate to us on a very personal level when we are dealing with pain and grief.

As you face future storms, I pray that you can take some encouragement from this to help you, by the grace of God, to make it through. I also pray that as the Lord proves Himself faithful to you, you will remember where the glory and praise is due, and that you will point the glory back to the Lord!

To God be the Glory for all He has done in and through my life!

— *Kristy Geiser*

I feel a responsibility with this book beyond sharing my story. Going through these storms has strengthened our faith, rather than weakened it. I see clearly now that, though we don't always have the choice of what storms come into our lives, we do have the choice of how we let them affect us. You've chosen to walk with me through our journey up to this point, and I invite you to continue one step further. I would like to share with you my personal beliefs about how you can also have a relationship with my Savior, as well as find strength in the specific places I still find strength today.

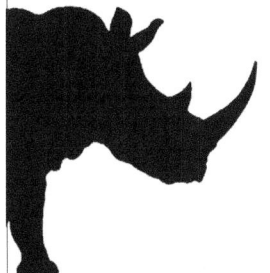

Epilogue: My Personal Message

Epilogue: My Personal Message

I would be remiss not to include in this book how you can have a personal relationship with the Lord Jesus Christ. I cannot imagine going through any type of trial without having Him by my side! Knowing that God Himself, the Creator of the universe, is there with me through it all, and realizing the fact that He has a will and a purpose for my life, helps all of the trials make sense.

I am thankful that I know the truth. He has proven His love for each and every one of us, and God's Word says He desires a relationship with us. He has shown me that He is real. He loves us and sent His Son to die on the cross for our sins. The best news is that we can know for *sure* that we are saved and going to Heaven. We can know that we will spend eternity with Jesus, our Savior. Through our salvation, we can escape hell, the devil, and an everlasting separation from God. The plan of salvation is simple, and anyone can be saved by the grace of God.

God is loving. I John 4:8 tells us that "God is love." Because of this, many would argue that He couldn't send anyone to hell, but that is not true. Psalm 9:16-17 says, "The Lord is known by the judgment which he executeth: the wicked is snared in the work of his own hands...The wicked shall be turned into hell, and all the nations that forget God." Not only is God loving, but He is also *just* and *holy*. Because He is just and holy, He must require sinless perfection in order to be in His presence. Because He cannot look upon sin, our sin separates us from Him.

First of all, we must recognize that we are sinners. There is not a single person who has not sinned. Sure, there are many who think of themselves as good people. They may be according to man's standards, but they are not judging themselves by God's standard. God gave us standards (commandments) in His Word that tell us what it takes to be holy. We all are guilty of many, if not all, of them. Romans 3:10-11, 23 says, "As it is written, There is none righteous, no, not one: There is none that

Epilogue: My Personal Message

understandeth, there is none that seeketh after God...For all have sinned, and come short of the glory of God."

Which person has never been disobedient to his parents? Who has not stolen anything? And which of us has never told a lie, even a small one, or even an untrue statement of sarcasm? What about taking the Lord's name in vain? The list goes on, and I know beyond a shadow of a doubt that we all are guilty of sinning against the God of Heaven. How can I say that so dogmatically? Because God's Word says that we are all sinners. "For ALL have sinned."

Romans 6:23 tells us of our fate as sinners, "For the wages of sin is death." Sin brings death. That is the only outcome of sin. "Death" means dying and being separated from God for eternity. There is no other possibility if we die in our sins.

We have to accept that we are sinners and on our way to hell. Hell is an eternal lake of fire where suffering and pain will be completely inescapable for all eternity! Hebrews 9:27 says, "And as it is appointed unto men once to die, but after this the judgment." Revelation 20:10, 12-15 says, "And the devil that deceived them was cast into the lake of fire and brimstone... and shall be tormented day and night forever and ever. And I saw the dead, small and great, stand before God, and the books were opened; and another book was opened, which is the book of life. And the dead were judged out of those things which were written in the books, according to their works...and they were judged every man according to their works. And whosoever was not found written in the book of life was cast into the lake of fire." These are literal words, not just fables, parables, and legends.

But God loves us so much, even in our sin, that He made a way of escape. We can have our name written in the Lamb's Book of Life! Romans 5:8 says, "But God commendeth his love toward us in that, while we were yet sinners, Christ died for us." Even when we were in an unlovely state, blackened and filthy with sin, God loved us enough to make a way of escape so we could live with Him for eternity. Romans 6:23 goes on to say, "But the gift of God is eternal life through Jesus Christ our Lord."

John 3:16-17 tells us, "For God so loved the world, that he gave his only begotten Son, that whosoever believeth in him should not perish, but have everlasting life. For God sent not his Son into the world to condemn the world, but that the world through him might be saved."

What do we need to do in order to be saved from our sins? Romans 10:9-10, 13 tells us, "That if thou shalt confess with thy mouth the Lord Jesus, and shalt believe in thine heart that God hath raised him from the dead, thou shalt be saved. For with the heart man believeth unto righteousness; and with the mouth confession is made unto salvation. For whosoever shall call upon the name of the Lord shall be saved." Confession has the meaning that we admit our sins and have the attitude of repentance. Repentance is changing our mind and agreeing with God's view of sin and Jesus' provision on Calvary. If we repent of our sins and put our faith and trust in Him, we will be saved. It is as simple as that.

God has promised to forgive our sins. We just have to ask for forgiveness! He is faithful, and He is just. Our sins can be completely washed away by the blood of Christ! Psalm 103:12 promises, "As far as the east is from the west, so far hath he removed our transgressions from us." Hebrews 8:12 continues that thought, "For I will be merciful to their unrighteousness, and their sins and their iniquities will I remember no more."

Luke 15:7 shows us the joy that is in Heaven when one comes to know the Lord, "I say unto you that likewise joy shall be in heaven over one sinner that repenteth." It is not God's will for any of us to die in our sins according to II Peter 3:9 which states, "The Lord is not slack concerning his promise, as some men count slackness, but is long-suffering toward us-ward, not willing that any should perish, but that all should come to repentance." It is God's desire and design that we come to Him for forgiveness and live in a close relationship with Him. These desires are clearly described in the scriptures.

Yet, many would argue that "religion is what we make of it, and what works for you might not work for me, but neither one is wrong." Truth is truth and there is no room in truth for adaptation. Even the slightest element of untruth in a statement makes the entire statement false. Truth is absolute.

Society teaches us to be tolerant of everyone's religious views, claiming that no one can dogmatically say that their "religion" is the only right one. We are being taught that truth is a perception, and in one person's perception of reality, the truth may be different than the truth in another's perception of reality. This destructive, yet popular, view is being taught by schools across the country.

I heard a brief interview of a college student who could not tell his interviewer that he was wrong when he said that two plus two equals seven. He said that seven could be correct in the interviewer's perception of reality. Even though he agreed that two plus two is four, he would not admit that the man he was talking to was wrong in saying that two plus two equals seven.

Having this mindset gives freedom to make poor decisions in a life free of guilt. It leaves no accountability for one's actions. If I make a decision that would be wrong for you, but it is right in my mind, then who are you to say that it is wrong? This mindset is both dangerous and destructive.

Removing absolute truth is destructive. Satan's ploy is to brainwash people into believing there is no such thing as right and wrong. If there is no absolute truth, then how can one say definitively that it is wrong to hurt someone? Or how can one argue that it is wrong to steal something from someone else? When right and wrong are left up to the conscience of each person, or lack thereof, the result is a downward spiral leading to an unstable and unsafe society. The book of Judges is full of examples where people would "do that which was right in their own eyes." This only led to the demise or destruction of that group through slavery, judgments, or death. There is no hope without truth.

I John 2:21-23 warns us, "I have not written unto you

because ye know not the truth, but because ye know it, and that no lie is of the truth. Who is a liar but he that denieth that Jesus is the Christ? He is antichrist, that denieth the Father and the Son. Whosoever denieth the Son, the same hath not the Father; he that acknowledgeth the Son hath the Father also." There are many false teachers who do not teach that Jesus Christ is God's Son. If Jesus Christ is not taught as God, the religion is false, period.

Many children are taught in school not to decide hastily about religion; they should hear all the ideas of different religions and then decide which one works for them—regardless of deciphering which one teaches truth. They can't *all* be right—that goes against all logic and reason. These children need to be taught that there *is* absolute truth and that only the Word of God can offer this truth.

If a religion teaches that you can be "saved," yet continue in your sin, the religion is false. This view of "salvation" is destructive and gives a false hope of eternal security in Heaven. True salvation naturally brings change—repentance is the key. II Corinthians 5:17 says, "Therefore if any man be in Christ, he is a new creature: old things are passed away; behold, all things are become new."

The Bible is the source of truth. It has been tried and tested, and it is the only book that has stood the test of time. There are too many fulfilled prophecies and proven facts given in the Bible for it not to be true. God has kept His Word pure as He has promised. Matthew 5:18 says, "Till heaven and earth pass, one jot or one tittle shall in no wise pass from the law, till all be fulfilled." Luke 16:17 agrees, "And it is easier for heaven and earth to pass, than one tittle of the law to fail." God is the Creator of the universe, and He is the author of all truth.

Some argue that they need reason and logic to come to Christ. But ultimately, there has to be the element of *faith*—believing in God. Therefore, accepting the truths of God's Word will be easier for some than for others. My hope and prayer is that if you do not have your eternity settled in Heaven, you will come to a saving knowledge of the Lord Jesus Christ today. You can have the wonderful assurance that if you were to die tonight, you could be absolutely sure that you would go to Heaven.

So many blessings come from living a life with God on your side. Romans 8:32 tells us, "He that spared not his own Son, but delivered him up for us all, how shall he not with him also freely give us all things?" Psalm 84:11 promises, "The Lord will give grace and glory. No good thing will he withhold from them that walk uprightly." I am in no way promoting the prosperity gospel that many are teaching today. I am not saying that once you're saved, the rest of your life will be free of storms; but I am saying that God is the One that can turn all things, including storms, into positive events in our lives. He can be glorified through our lives, even through negative circumstances.

Through salvation, our relationship with the Lord is permanent. You can never lose your salvation. Romans 8:35, 37-39 promises, "Who shall separate us from the love of Christ? Shall tribulation, or distress, or persecution, or famine, or nakedness, or peril, or sword? Nay, in all these things we are more than conquerors through him that loved us. For I am persuaded that neither death, nor life, nor angels, nor principalities, nor powers, nor things present, nor things to come, nor height, nor depth, nor any other creature, shall be able to separate us from the love of God, which is in Christ Jesus, our Lord." Once we are saved, nothing in this world can separate us from God! We can go through storms knowing that God will be there with us through it all.

I trust that the Lord will use this book in your life as you continue on life's journey. I hope that as you encounter future trials, you may remember many of the concepts and truths in this book to help you through.

I pray that the one thing you take from this book is the importance of first having a relationship with the Lord. Secondly, you rely on that relationship for the grace, comfort, and blessings that are so readily available through the valleys of life. I have been on the mountain top as well as in the valley, and I can say with one-hundred percent certainty that God is good even in the valley! I'd even dare say that God is good *especially* in the valleys. All the praise, honor, and glory belong to the Lord for His grace and love in my life!

Resources

The Bible

Financial Help
www.daveramsey.com

St. Jude Children's Research Hospital
www.stjude.org

Spiritual Guidance
www.thewayofthemaster.com

Discipleship
www.fbcsantamaria.com

Acknowledgments

Special thanks to Adam Tillinghast for his tireless help and work on this book.

Special thanks to Kelly Ferreira Photography for the incredible photos of our family over the years, many of which were used throughout this book.

The balloon shown in picture on page 116 used with permission of Suzy's Zoo, © Suzy Spafford.

www.ingramcontent.com/pod-product-compliance
Lightning Source LLC
Chambersburg PA
CBHW072335300426
44109CB00042B/1622